"The Invisible Fitness will inspire readers to heal the obstacle of body shame and claim a lifestyle of healthier eating and fitness as their authentic practice rather than merely following a fad."

Michael Bernard Beckwith
Author of *Life Visioning*

"I've been lucky to know and work with JJ for almost 20 years. She is the most passionate and knowledgeable trainer I've ever met. Her experience, insights, and excitement to make her clients stronger, healthier, and happier shows in her latest book. Do yourself a huge favor and start reading **The Invisible Fitness Formula: 5 Secrets to Release Weight and End Body Shame** today."

Heather Lounsbury, L.Ac.,
Author of *Fix Your Mood with Food*

"If you're like me, for most of my life, my inner battle with my body was brutal...even when I was twenty years old and weighed 120 pounds! As a dream expert, author, and hypnotherapist, my work with clients (and myself) has been all about the business of learning to have a love affair with the body we have. JJ Flizanes is an amazing teacher, leader, guide, and coach and her book, **The Invisible Fitness Formula: 5 Secrets to Release Weight and End Body Shame** is drenched in practical tips and the tools we all need to release body shame and awaken to the body of our dreams...no matter what size and shape that may be!"

Kelly Sullivan Walden
Bestselling Author of "The Love, Sex
& Relationship Dream Dictionary"

"*The Invisible Fitness Formula* is a comprehensive guide to total wellness. It clearly and concisely covers the bases of how to get fit and stay that way from a whole person perspective while identifying the root cause connected to weight gain and body shame. It should be used as a reference over and again for anyone that truly desires to transform their health and fitness levels. JJ Flizanes is thorough, insightful, highly knowledgeable, deep, and passionate about total wellness. This is a must read for your health!"

Dr. Meg Haworth

Author/Celebrity Chef/Holistic Wellness Expert

"I have worked with JJ for many years and know how sincerely she is committed to help her clients optimize their health on all levels. JJ's book is a rare combo of addressing many of the root causes of weight loss resistance and body shame. Writing in a user friendly style, she provides a comprehensive approach and a plan of action to help you deal with the core issues to awaken your vital health. I will be recommending her book to my patients."

Allen H. Peters MD Medical Director

Nourishing Wellness Medical Center

"I was one of those people who was exercising more and more while accomplishing less and less. I even spent three hours a day doing cardio, trying to lose weight for my upcoming wedding; but it wasn't until JJ enlightened me about what I was missing that I finally got results. By combing resistance training and reducing sugar and other carbs from my diet, I was able to lose 30 pounds with only a fraction of the effort. JJ's expertise outlined my path to healthy, sustainable weight loss – with an added and unexpected benefit of no more heartburn. I LOVE this book! *The Invisible Fitness Formula: 5 Secrets to Release Weight and End Body Shame* gave me more insights about what's going on in my diet and what I can do to keep improving my health Thank you, JJ, for sharing your wisdom in this indispensable book for anyone wanting to take back control of their health and weight."

Michael Neeley

Author of The Art of Forgetting and Host of Consciously Speaking

"If you are serious about making the changes you want to make, then there is no one more inspirational than JJ Flizanes. She is tenacious but kind, knowledgeable but not presumptive, informative in a highly intelligent way but encouraging with a sense of gentle equality, and empowering by her own "walking her talk." She embodies compassionate empowerment."

Valerie Maxwell, Ph.D., Psychologist

"As an energy worker and healer, what I find people struggle with the most is self acceptance, self love and self confidence. I love that not only does *The Invisible Fitness Formula* cover scientific secrets that can help us release weight, JJ Flizanes dives right into the emotional blocks that perpetuate body shame. This book will not only help our physical health, but it can be the way to heal what is really at the core. Bravo!"

Lisa Thomas, Beyond Cellular Healings

"As a makeover & confidence expert, I deal with people who struggle with their image, which negatively impacts the way they perceive themselves. JJ Flizanes completely nails the steps women can take to change their body image and consequently their confidence. *The Invisible Fitness Formula* will absolutely transform the way you look and feel holistically from the inside out. What I love about this book, is that it gives a hand-on and step-by-step approach in helping people get results. Bravo JJ... I will definitely be giving this to my clients!"

Kim Seltzer, Confidence & Makeover Expert/Therapist

"As someone who has struggled with eating around my digestion and autoimmune issues, JJ Flizanes has become an invaluable asset. I've learned so many easy, delicious recipes from her podcast and YouTube shows that have been pretty easy to recreate in my own kitchen. And we've enjoyed many paleo-friendly foods together – that can be found right in your local health food store. If you struggle with hormone-related inflammation, weight gain or illness, JJ's recipes and trainings are a must to help your body thrive."

Melanie Benson, Small Business Optimizer

"JJ Flizanes is a master at helping you change your relationship with yourself to put yourself first and then help you define specific self-care strategies that will work for you to experience the power to make choices that get you the results you want."

Dr. Lisa Galper, Power Over Food

"In our health and wellness world of many confusing messages, it can be overwhelming for someone looking for the right answers to let go of old weight and become the healthy person they were born to be. What I love and respect most about JJ is that she understands that our personal wellness is only realized once the body is congruent with the heart and mind. This is an incredible guide for both men and women to realize their potential, not only in their personal wellness, but in the ways they show up for themselves and for the people they care about. Coming from a weight loss of 75 pounds myself, I can relate to and emphasize with the feelings of shame. As JJ uncovers, shame is simply old programming from a story that doesn't serve us, and once we learn how to remove and replace, our lives can radically change from a place of true commitment and self-love. *The Invisible Fitness Formula* is a book for anyone that has made the decision to let go and move forward with their wellness.

Josh Trent, Host, Wellness Force Radio

"JJ is a powerful force in the wellness community. Her knowledge, passion and dedication are unparalleled. The body can heal itself if given the tools it needs to do so. JJ not only effortlessly guides us to understand how this is possible, but she also provides us the exact steps to take action in our own lives. JJ helps us let go of judgement, harsh regimens & old stories to embrace a new way of healing from the inside out. By loving ourselves and our bodies first, the true healing process can begin. A radical transformation of body, mind & spirit is possible and The Invisible Fitness Formula shows us the way."

Allison Melody, Host of Food Heals Podcast and
Author of The Healing Kitchen

"JJ offers you the opportunity and a method to discover what you truly want—body, mind, and spirit—and a way of fulfillment that lasts a lifetime. Imagine stepping into transformation and getting off that endless wheel of food and weight. Imagine nurturing your body and becoming the person you were always meant to be. Now there will be more of the inner you. Parts of yourself that you may not even have known. JJ's program is comprehensive and yet she manages to keep it simple enough for us to actually do."

Lorrie Kazan, Author of Happiness Calls Your Name

"As someone who is passionate about health, fitness and mindfulness, **The Invisible Fitness Formula** by JJ Flizanes has it all. This detailed book sizzles with knowledge backed with compelling evidence. With childhood obesity on the rise and food allergies rampant in our society, make no mistake it's time to make changes. It's clear that JJ is an advocate and is passionate that you achieve positive results. Take a look for yourself - I couldn't put it down."

Helen Hodgson, Author Couple's Massage Handbook - Deepen
Your Relationship with the Healing Power of Touch

*"**The Invisible Fitness Formula** is a must read book for anyone looking to create lasting weight loss **and** optimal health. I have known JJ for almost 20 years and she is a unique combination of expert fitness trainer, nutritionist and life coach with a profound understanding of the science of how the body works. She has put decades of know-how into an easy to read, comprehensive book that offers a holistic approach to weight loss and a path to create lasting health that applies to everyone. As someone who has dealt with auto-immune issues, I found the book filled with valuable information that address both the physical and emotional issues that underlie weight loss and other addictive behaviors. JJ gives us easy to use tools, information and resources that produce real world results. I am grateful for the gifts I have received from this book. "*

Adoley Odunton, Spiritual Life Coach,

Creator of the Wellness Revolution online series

"All too often we try and focus on only the macro parts of weight loss, mainly food and exercise, neglecting the most important part... What's going on inside of us. Stress, emotions, and our beliefs play a huge part in creating or undermining our health. JJ unpacks it all and makes it super simple to understand. **The Invisible Fitness Formula: 5 Secrets to Release Weight and End Body Shame** is a beautiful guide for creating real weight loss from the inside out. JJ really addresses weight loss and wellness from all angles, a true whole person approach, focused on loving yourself and feeling good. Know that when you are working with JJ, she leaves no stone unturned."

Jeff Agostinelli, The Next Level Podcast

"I have worked with trainers of many kinds over the years, but I will never forget my first training with JJ. I was astonished by the depth of her scientific knowledge; her ability to get to the heart of the matters I wanted to focus on; and the infinite tenderness and respect with which she treated me. I had never felt so clearly seen, heard, listened to and understood as I did - and do - with JJ. In reading *The Invisible Fitness Formula: 5 Secrets to Release Weight and End Body Shame,* I feel embraced once again by her deep humanity, caring and knowledge. I'm sure that you, the reader, will experience this too. This is one of those magical books that illuminate your understanding of yourself and why you've done what you've done - and gently guides you toward making new choices that bring results far beyond what you had in mind when you picked up this book in the first place. You will be delighted by who you become as you walk this path with JJ. And thank you JJ for loving us all enough to bring forth this book. It is amazing. You are amazing."

Moira Shepard, Transformational teacher

"*The Invisible Fitness Formula* is a revolution toward more health and vitality with compassion, soul-baring revelations and the kind of clarity that can take your breath away. The stage is set within the first few pages – stop buying the bullshit, give up deprivation and work the process from the inside-out. Concluding with powerful stories from clients, this book spoke to me as a life-long 'curvy' to 'beaudacious' (and back again) woman. I have read the books, done the programs, joined the gyms, hired the trainers – I even became a consultant for a weight loss food program (and became the only consultant to gain 10 lbs!). So I've 'been there, done it' and was a bit skeptical that I would learn anything new. To my surprise, I found this book to be spiritual salve with physical how-tos included (vs. the tradition approach being the other way around); it was easy to consume and, even more importantly, I wanted to read it. In short, my defenses were disarmed and my spirit engaged. I highly recommend this book to anyone who has exhausted the gamut of resource but still wants better health and vitality. (And now I'm off to practice positive thinking while I walk!)"

Lynn Scheurell, Creative Catalyst

"JJ is a passionate expert who can help you transform your life. She understands that changing your body image is about far more than food and exercise; it is about your whole person, including mindset, personal beliefs, and repressed fears. JJ understands why we often continue to live out our patterns, unwilling to be vulnerable enough to ask for help. She knows that we frequently surround ourselves with people who tell us what we want to hear because of inner beliefs telling us we are not enough. ***The Invisible Fitness Formula: 5 Secrets to Release Weight and End Body Shame*** is devoted to helping others become healthier and happier, as JJ communicates her vast knowledge with clarity in an easy-to-understand format. Feel her energy,experience and attitude and you'll be inspired to implement real change into your life."

Bruce Langford, Host of the Mindfulness Mode Podcast

"**The Invisible Fitness Formula** is a refreshing take on fi and weight loss without the shaming that so often comes within the industry. JJ's holistic approach addresses the underlying causes of not only weight gain, but also fatigue and other related health issues. JJ not only shares sound nutrition and exercise approaches, but also addresses the emotional elements that get in the way of making healthier choices. As someone who has personally dealt with adrenal fatigue and related weight most of my adult life, JJ's book comes at just the right time! JJ is a gifted woman if I ever met one and I highly recommend her book!"

Aurora Remember Holtzman

Host of Embracing Intensity Podcast

"JJ's passion for health and fitness is apparent in her holistic approach that includes both physical and emotional well-being through customized nutrition, exercise and mindfulness. She's an expert in her field, detail oriented, intuitive yet analytical and delivers the best possible solution to fit her clients' needs. Most importantly, JJ's programs are rooted in her determination, integrity and compassion setting the foundation for her clients' success in reaching their health and fitness goals."

Homa Sajadian Sikon, L.Ac., Dipl.Ac.

"JJ has an infectious smile and an energy that lights up any room. This may sound impossible but she actually makes me want to work out and be healthy because she has such a positive attitude and approach. She effortlessly makes me view it as a lifestyle and she challenges me every day!

Robert E. Blackmon, Author, designer and lifestyle expert

"JJ knows fitness and our health and happiness is what she's all about. She infuses heart and soul into our fitness regimen, which propels us from a more meaningful place, the result being fitness habits that stick, and that integrate into our daily lives, showing us that it CAN be done."

Julie Ferman, Matchmaker & Dating Coach

THE INVISIBLE FITNESS FORMULA

5 Secrets to Release Weight & End Body Shame

JJ Flizanes

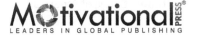

M⊙tivationalPRESS®
LEADERS IN GLOBAL PUBLISHING

Published by Motivational Press, Inc.
1777 Aurora Road
Melbourne, Florida, 32935
www.MotivationalPress.com

Copyright 2017 © by JJ Flizanes
Photo credit: Starla Fortunato (back cover image)

Manufactured in the United States of America.

ISBN: 978-1-62865-406-6

CONTENTS

Acknowledgments. 18
Foreword. 20
Introduction 23

CHAPTER 1 32
Divorcing the Scale
CHAPTER 2 41
New Habits Don't Fix the Problem
CHAPTER 3 47
Secret 1: Heal Digestion
CHAPTER 4 59
Elimination Diets
CHAPTER 5 65
Understanding Sugar
CHAPTER 6 72
Why Paleo
CHAPTER 7 80
Secret 2: Get Smart Exercise
CHAPTER 8 93
Build the Program
CHAPTER 9 102
Secret 3: Balance and Replenish Hormones
CHAPTER 10 114
The Orchestra of Sex Hormones
CHAPTER 11. 125
Additional Important Markers
CHAPTER 12 135
Secret 4: Embracing & Processing Feelings
CHAPTER 13 143
The Anatomy of Emotion
CHAPTER 14 153
How To Stop Shaming Yourself
CHAPTER 15 159
Secret 5: The Courage To Connect

What People Are Saying. 171
About the Author 194
Resources & References 196
References 200

First, I dedicate this book to every Invisible Fitness client I have ever worked with, personally, over the last twenty years. Your trust has fueled a burning desire in me to help solve your problem situations and be relentless in the pursuit of what the "truth" and the "root" was for each and every one of you. Thank you for inspiring me to keep learning and for trusting me to be your guide.

Second, I dedicate this book to every listener of The Fit 2 Love Podcast Show. During the first 2 seasons and 340 shows, your feedback, patronage, and excitement about the show allowed me to know that I was on the right track.

Lastly, but not least, I also dedicate this book to my husband, Brian Albers and my parents Gus and Valerie Flizanes. Every show and every word has you in mind. Not only do I want to inspire, educate, and heal the world, but what I want most is for you to be the happiest and healthiest you can be so I can enjoy my time on this earth with you as long as possible. I love you.

ACKNOWLEDGMENTS

I HAVE TO START OFF with the two biggest contributors to the information I have learned over the last ten years- Dr. Allen Peters and Jeanne Peters. I could not have written this book without you. Working with Nourishing Wellness and being part of the team has not only helped my clients with their health, but mine too! I love you both and appreciate that our relationship is personal as well as professional.

Thanks to Dr. Elizabeth Plourde, whose own health struggle became the catalyst for her extensive hormone research. I support your passion for getting the truth out there.

Thank you Lynne Boutross for sharing your wisdom, gifts of sight, and intuition. You have helped me see more clearly and I hope our work will help more people do the same.

Thank you to Rodger Sorrow and the late Dr. Marshall Rosenberg for **Non Violent Communication**. I know this work can change the world and bring peace and joy to every person who masters it; my life is better because of it.

Thank you to Jack Barnard for branding Invisible Fitness so many years ago - you are a master of branding. I could never have guessed what a perfect umbrella it would be for the last fifteen years of my growth and expansion.

Thank you to Mark and Bibi Goldstein for allowing me to use your home to start the creative process.

Thank you Trent and Olga Jones for the refuge in Ojai, as well as your lovely beach home retreat where much of this came together. I appreciate your support!

Thank you to Lisa Thomas for helping to unlock some of the creative juices and clear stuck energy to allow this to come through.

To Susan Grady, Julie Wolf, Echo Allen, Macarena Bianchi, Jeanne Peters and my 30 Day Manifestation Challenge Group who supported my daily appreciation for every step of this journey. I love the tribe we are building and I look forward to expanding that into this work too.

To Gus and Valerie Flizanes for the endless support you always provide me. I could not have better parents and I am grateful for you every day. I love you, thank you!

Finally, to my hero, my husband Brian Albers, thank you for being a great provider of everything during this process. You have been a super star and I appreciate you. Thank you H, I love you!!

FOREWORD

IF YOU'VE STRUGGLED with finding a deeper, healthier, and happier connection to your body, food, and lifestyle, this book may be your bible. Recent research in mind –body medicine indicates that if we are truly going to heal the obesity epidemic that has tripled in the past fifty years, a holistic, mindful approach is key.

As a Registered Dietitian, along with my husband, an integrative doctor, we co-founded the Nourishing Wellness Medical Center to help men and women feel more vital by balancing their hormones, body chemistry, and improving metabolism through healthier food/ lifestyle/exercise choices and other natural therapies. Our work models what change is possible through an integrative approach that addresses the root cause of obesity and disease.

This is how we came to appreciate the work of JJ Flizanes. She was hired as our Exercise Specialist to develop a sustainable exercise programs for our clients. She impressed us with her knowledge of anatomy, physiology, physics, and biomechanics to develop a personalized exercise program that was effective in building muscle, burning fat, and improving balance but preserved joint integrity. To this day, JJ continues to work with several clients who have completely eliminated pain within 6 months of her guidance and continue to gain benefit after a decade of her services.

After witnessing JJ's work with our clients for many years, I can truly say she is a gifted coach and motivator. She has an almost mystic-like capacity to understand complex problems and issues related to the body/mind connection and to explain them succinctly in a language and style that inspires her clients towards action. She is also a wonderful, caring friend and a kindred spirit for me personally. We have that kind of relationship where I can talk with her about almost anything for hours.

JJ's book *The Invisible Fitness Formula: 5 Secrets to Release Weight and End Body Shame* is so timely and important. Her desire is help you understand the invisible forces at play that impact the visible aspects of your body and health. Authentic sustainable change must come from within and JJ will help you identify your core limiting beliefs that are keeping you stuck with your weight. You'll discover ways to transform your negative thoughts and feelings that drain your energy and replace them with positive thoughts that empower you to love, accept and take better care of your body. You will feel JJ's message fl w from her heart to yours when you read her personal struggles with body shame and how she transformed this pain into deep acceptance. She uses her stories to help change the conversation about body image, dieting, and what has been proven to help solve this crisis.

JJ's chapter on Heal Digestion makes a positive contribution to understanding the connection between the quality of our food choices and its influence on the health of our gut. For example, recent research has shown that our gut flora can improve our weight loss, our health, and even our moods. JJ encourages you to delve deeper into the role of food sensitivities and discover how this may play a role in your symptoms such as belly bloat, constipation, mood swings, and inflammation. She offers some practical steps on how to eat to help heal your gut lining and improve your digestive function.

She debunks common myths in her chapter on exercise, such as "the best way to lose weight is to exercise more". She explains the power in knowing your target heart rate so you design an exercise routine to be more efficient with your time. She reveals the shortcomings in excessive cardio for weight loss and explains how to optimize your metabolism through mindfulness during strength training.

Sharing success stories from her clients, JJ explains the value of working from the inside out when it comes to your relationship to food. You'll discover the effect that food and stress have on your hormones like insulin and cortisol. You'll discover ways to listen to the body and guide your food choices towards quality and pleasure while eating. These practices can further enhance digestion, hormones, and your metabolism. This is the way to true health.

True health is not just about the weight you release, it's about the life you gain in the process. If you follow JJ's secrets to re-program the body and mind from the inside out, you will discover how to release the body shame and the weight you no longer need, while you learn how to care for the body you have. It's time for a fresh new holistic approach to living lean and attracting greater health and well-being. Start with reading this book and pay attention- there is so much to learn here!

Jeanne Peters RD Nutrition Director
Nourishing Wellness Medical Center
Redondo Beach, CA

INTRODUCTION

"We get to decide for ourselves what is beautiful
when it comes to our bodies ."

Jennifer Aniston

IN 1996, I DECIDED to pursue an education in personal training. Working in the gym as a receptionist, I found myself attracted to how strong the female body could look. However, it wasn't about just the "outside", I was drawn towards how I interpreted that would feel.

Since the beginning, I have been learning about science and how to apply it to our bodies to make changes and improvements. Every step of the way, my respect for the human body deepened as I learned more. After learning about biomechanics, I was even factoring in the longevity of my joints and I was barely in my twenties.

Through biomechanics, anatomy, physiology, biochemistry, and physics, I have come to have a profound regard for my body for the miracle and perfection that it is. The more I learn, the more I love my body.

Now I am not saying I love the way it always looks on the outside, I am in an industry that quickly judges the way you look and uses it to determine how much you know. Talk about judging a book by its cover! Part of the motivation to get into this work was to improve my relationship with how my body looked on the outside too.

Puberty happened early for me, around age thirteen, and since I was one of the only girls in class with hips and breasts, I felt ugly.

I was even a cheerleader in junior high and was considered a "base" because I had hips that someone could use as "stairs" to climb onto my shoulders. All the skinny girls were able to be on the top while I knew from the beginning I was too heavy and too curvy at this point to ever experience that.

I was not considered a pretty girl in high school either, so I know what it's like to feel shame for your body and feel invisible among a sea of hormonal teenagers. Yet, I know that feeling awkward and ugly helped to strengthen my self-esteem because I was forced to focus on other aspects of my talent and intelligence. I have met many beautiful people through the years that carry more insecurity and shame because their looks have always been what they perceived to be their biggest asset.

In my last book, *Fit 2 Love: How to Get Physically, Emotionally, and Spiritually Fit to Attract the Love of Your Life*, I introduced the "love yourself first" concept because it had been my experience. I manifested my husband because I chose to love myself first and get my own needs met instead of feeling as if I was missing something because I didn't have a partner.

Every day is still a practice for me to decide to love and accept myself as I am and stop comparing myself to other fitness celebrities who are more fit or attractive. It's not easy to put yourself out there in this way and to be judged.

I have had to learn, and keep practicing, to radically and

unapologetically love, and accept myself while I put myself out into the world center stage, vulnerably exposed to all kinds of judgement and opinion. When I talk about shame, I have experienced it firsthand my whole life. I am faced with it every day that I do my job and business. I have made peace with my body, my purpose, and I repeatedly chose love over popularity.

Because I've also rebelled against my industry's narcissistic need to focus on every pound and every inch of muscle definition, or lack of it, this makes me a different kind of trainer.

I am highly sensitive to shaming, I do my best to make sure my actions, and words are being received with the love and support I intend. I avoid people who I may know are struggling because I can feel the tension when I am around, as if I am judging them- I stay away, so they don't feel nervous or confronted.

I feel uncomfortable when I run into someone who has lost weight because it puts me in an awkward position. If I acknowledge their weight loss, I might be adding power to a belief that you are only beautiful when you are thinner.

However, if I do not say anything, I might come across as if I don't care. I care about your health but I care more that you get your results from respecting your body and making choices that support your systems.

I don't really care what you look like I care how you feel. I care that you made the choice not to eat the pasta because you know it will cause damage to your digestion. I don't support that you feel restricted and only avoided it because it is high in calories and could cause weight gain.

I was a guest coach on a 90-Day weight loss challenge, and during the 12-week program, I never asked my team how much weight they lost. Towards the end, I asked them if they had noticed that I never asked them each week how much weight they lost. They did notice and I asked, "Do you know why I don't ask you? It's because I do not want to strengthen the idea that your self-worth or success has anything to do with a number. I don't count calories or track a number on a scale and I don't believe it supports your self-acceptance. This just reinforces the ideas that we all rebel against, whether you are aware of it or not, that your self-worth has anything to do with the scale.

My mission is to change the conversation. We are already talking about it but we need to include every man, woman, and child who feels less than beautiful or attractive because they do not look like someone in the media.

One of my favorite actresses, Jennifer Aniston, recently published an article in the **Huffington Post** that really spoke to this growing need in our society to change the conversation.

She was being emotionally pushed over the edge with relentless attention to her body and speculations of whether or not she was pregnant. Her article was published on The Huffington Post website on July 12th 2016 titled "For the Record".

"If I am some kind of symbol to some people out there, then clearly I am an example of the lens through which we, as a society, view our mothers, daughters, sisters, wives, female friends and colleagues. The objectification and scrutiny we put women through is absurd and disturbing. The way I am portrayed by the media is simply a reflection of how we see and portray women in general, measured against some warped standard of beauty. Sometimes cultural standards just need a different perspective so we can see them for what

they really are — a collective acceptance... a subconscious agreement. We are in charge of our agreement. Little girls everywhere are absorbing our agreement, passive or otherwise. And it begins early. The message that girls are not pretty unless they're incredibly thin, that they're not worthy of our attention unless they look like a supermodel or an actress on the cover of a magazine is something we're all willingly buying into. This conditioning is something girls then carry into womanhood. ..."...

Jennifer goes on to address how the media plays a significant role in creating body shame and how both celebrities and the average person has been affected by this. I was so moved by the article that I wanted to share some of it here and encourage everyone to read it on The Huffington Post website. At the end, she encourages us to take specific action collectively to shift this paradigm.

"...From years of experience, I've learned tabloid practices, however dangerous, will not change, at least not any time soon. What can change is our awareness and reaction to the toxic messages buried within these seemingly harmless stories served up as truth and shaping our ideas of who we are. We get to decide how much we buy into what's being served up, and maybe some day the tabloids will be forced to see the world through a different, more humanized lens because consumers have just stopped buying the bullshit."

Amen.

Will you join us in changing the conversation? In order to do that, you must decide that you are valuable and worthy as you are right now, and that any decision you make when it comes to your body will be made from a place of love and respect and no longer from shame and self-loathing.

We have to be brave and courageous to accept ourselves as we are right now. When we continue the concept of "I will be happy when I get to the weight I want" or "I will like myself when...." we perpetuate this illusion that there is an external standard that controls our happiness. As Jennifer Aniston said above, in order for this to change, we have to stop "buying the bullshit". Giving power to these ideas of beauty and perfection will always keep us victimized and disempowered.

MY COMMITMENT TO YOU

This work and everything I do, is about empowering you. I believe in you, and I believe in your ability to heal and release that which no longer serves you.

The information and tools that are inside this book are keys to achieving the body, health, and happiness level you desire.

Too often, the ideas of fitness and weight loss are served up with an extra-large helping of shame and guilt because you have been told that it is will power alone that drives your choices and therefore your results. So you feel like a failure when you "fall off the wagon". You think you "should" have been able to muscle your way through it with mental determination alone. You might feel that you are not strong enough mentally and that couldn't be further from the truth.

While we are going to take a medical and scientific approach and look at all the factors on a physical level, we are also going to take a deep dive into your soul. One of the most misunderstood ideas about habits is their emotional root. Just like weeding a garden, if you cut or break the weed at the top it will just grow back. In order to eliminate it completely, you must dig down and pull it out at the root.

While reading this will inevitably lead to greater awareness of factors you may have missed or overlooked, this is a process. Be gentle and kind to yourself. There is a lot to do but I also want you to balance out the *"do-ing"* with *"be-ing"*.

There is no end point- we are always evolving and expanding. You are right where you need to be, in perfect timing. There is a reason we are meeting at this place on your journey.

I am here to lay out the process and then gently guide you through it. Pretend you know nothing about your body, health, or weight loss. Clean the slate and be open to a new way of looking at your body and this journey. We will start with simple concepts and ideas first so you can implement them right away and see results.

The Invisible Fitness brand is about incorporating everything visible and invisible. The invisible forces at play that effect every aspect of your health from your joints, hormones, digestion, and stress level are equally if not more important than the aspects of your body that you can see.

Over the years, Invisible Fitness has expanded into including the invisible forces of your emotions, mind, and spirit. The more you embrace the power of your emotions, the faster you will experience transformation as we go through these steps. Many people give lip service to stress and then go on to ignore its strong presence in their daily lives, never addressing the real issues and continue sabotaging patterns that keep them stuck exactly where they've been for years.

There is not one system in the body that works alone- each part affects the whole. The reason you may not have found lasting success with releasing weight or improving health to this point is because you have been missing key pieces in that puzzle.

Within these pages, you will get everything you need to empower your success. Step-by-step, implement each piece and allow it to integrate into your life before moving onto the next step. I have even developed a 5 month program that can help you implement each step and keep you accountable along the way for true transformation.

Listen to your intuition at each stage, and know that this blueprint is the foundation that you will keep returning back to as you age and your lifestyle changes. The principles and steps will not change but your relationship to the work will. Your body will require different applications of these steps as you age. Your emotional health will need different tools as you heal and clear away patterns and old, stuck energy.

I have been utilizing these steps with clients, family, and myself for the past ten years. As I moved into a new stage of life over the last few years, I too needed to go back and address each one of these steps.

Take a deep breath and trust that life is working out for you. Trust that this information has made its way into your hands because you are now ready for it. Congratulate yourself for having the courage to move forward. Do the work and forgive yourself for any unrealistic expectations that you have had up to this point.

HOW TO START

If you are a left brained, structured person, you may want to do an evaluation of where you are now to determine what step to focus on implementing first. You can take a short assessment at fit2love.tv/quiz that will help you identify the gaps in your current or past programs.

You may want to take some measurements, if you are someone who is motivated by numbers, but I caution you to do this once and then put away the scale for at least three months. While in this book I will encourage you to try new things and create new habits, I will also be encouraging you to release the habits that no longer serve you-and the scale is the first one.

CHAPTER 1

DIVORCING THE SCALE

"The beauty of a woman is not in the clothes she wears, the figure that she carries or the way she combs her hair ."

Audrey Hepburn

I F WE ARE TO OVERCOME body shaming, we have to divorce the scale. There is no greater action that invalidates our sense of self-worth faster than that number.

Are you one of those people who gets on the scale every morning or every day to see how you're going to feel about yourself? If you answered yes, this is a problem. The scale may be keeping you stuck.

Don't you know people who count calories and get on the scale all the time, yet they haven't changed their body at all? Or they go up and down 10 or 15 pounds, but never really keep it off and it's a constant cycle? The scale is not the answer.

Let's review all the physiological as well as psychological reasons why the scale is not the best measurement of what's going on in your body.

First, it's not the only measure.

Most people get on the scale to see whether or not it has increased or decreased which then gets translated into *"I've lost weight"* or *"I've gained weight."* From that point, many people feel either, happy or sad depending on which way it went.

Those emotions have now colored the rest of your day. Then the self-talk *(or self-abuse)* after what's happened on the scale is vulnerable to whatever those feelings are that come up, and the judgment that comes up about what has happened or went wrong.

First, and foremost, the scale measures your entire mass. That consists of your bones, blood, organs, muscle, fat, the water in you (which is greater than 70% of your body weight), anything left over in your digestive system, your hair, skin, and nails.

Your mass is every single thing that makes up your body composition. Notice in that list of body composition that fat was only *one of the components.* When you step on the scale, people are looking for "how much fat did I gain or lose?" The scale can't tell you that.

Now, there are scales that do body fat composition. While I think that the better brands are good to have, the idea of going to the scale in order to see if you've lost or gained some fat is an act of giving up power and being completely susceptible to the interpretation of that number.

There are three places from where you can gain or lose weight: muscle, fat, and water. However, the scale will not be able to tell you which one of those has changed.

If it's water, then it can probably be easily lost as fast as it was gained. There are many components that effect why we hold on to water, such as if you had an extra salty meal or you ate some gluten or dairy. Let's say you've had some dairy and you're now constipated. You just haven't eliminated the food that's in your body. Sometimes having a proper elimination can help to release some of the water and some of that extra weight that you're seeing on the scale.

If you eat gluten, dairy, and have inflammatory foods like sugars in your diet, you're going to have a spike in your weight gain quickly because of the amount of water your body has to hold on to with those foods; because those foods cause internal inflammation .

If you're looking at that number as an indication of how well you're doing, it really can't tell you that. I have had clients who have lost 3% body fat and 3 inches around their waist while the scale stayed exactly the same.

The illusion that the scale creates will also incorrectly validate what you have been doing. If you have been the same weight for 10 years without resistance training, you probably think you are doing a good job. But in that 10-year period, you have lost 15 pounds of muscle and have gained 15 pounds of fat.

Even though the number on the scale is exactly the same, your body composition has changed. What that means is as you creep up in age, year after year, your metabolism is slower than it was last year. Over time, if the exercise becomes less and the food stays the same, you're more susceptible for weight gain. Then it will be harder to lose it in the future when your metabolism is slower. I can't stress enough that the scale is not a good reading for body composition or giving you a full picture about what's happening in your body.

Let's redefine the relationship with the scale. Why do you even step on it in the first place? What's at the bottom of your desire to lose weight? Is it to be healthier and to live longer? Or is it to be happier and to feel good?

Imagine yourself at the exact body weight and body shape that you desire. How do you feel? What comes up for you? What do you tell yourself you're going to feel when you get to the destination that you have in your mind?

I'm going to guess that you think you will feel better and accept yourself. You're going to feel more confident. It all comes back to being happier and more confident, which you can do without losing weight. In fact, it's my belief that you have to do that before you **can** lose weight. You can be happy and feel good now. In fact, you cause resistance to weight loss when you demand that your body change first before you accept it as it is now.

The energy that surrounds judging yourself, when you're beating yourself up for not losing weight or for being where you are, is almost like having a friend who you're yelling at, and then you expect them to do what you're asking of them. If you want your friend to tell you that you look nice today, but yet you're telling them that they're not good enough, that they look ugly, and that they're dressed poorly today, they probably won't turn around and be nice to you because of the energy you're putting out to them.

The rejection of your body creates an energy that your body wants to rebel against because you're shaming it.

The number on the scale can mask some really important information such as the fact that your metabolism is slowing down. Catch that early, and you can add some resistance training and build muscle, so that you don't lose active tissue in order to maintain or even increase your metabolism.

What happens too often, especially with women, is that there's zero resistance training going on. There is zero paying attention to the body fat composition. Then around age 47- 55, there is this quick weight gain, and then this shock about "Well, I was exercising. I was doing cardio, and my food hasn't changed. What happened?" What happened was, for 10 or 20 years, your metabolism was slowly decreasing because of hormonal decrease with no effort in building muscle to preserve your metabolism.

Many people think shaming themselves with a scale will keep them in line and hyper-focused on eating less calories or trying to fit in some exercise. While that may sound like a good way to do it, it backfires because you feel restricted and the body feels disrespected. You're really not happy because you're living in such a small box of what you're able to do. This isn't a lifestyle change. This is almost like being chained up because you don't feel free. When you don't feel free, you can't feel happy.

You've given all your power over to the scale and this almost random number, so inevitably you feel trapped. The beliefs and feelings of inadequacy, not being good enough, and not feeling confident about your body then get anchored even deeper into your subconscious and continue the pattern, which keeps you starting a new program every year.

Even if you're on a successful weight loss program right now that has you counting calories, watching what you eat, and exercising, you need to understand that the root of all of this *isn't just the food*. There's a reason why you choose to use food to satisfy a need and to feel relief. We will be exploring this deeper, later in the program, but let me plant the seed now so by the time we get there, you are ready to take a good look at your beliefs and emotions.

Another reason why the scale is detrimental is that it keeps supporting the abuse and disrespect of where you are now. If you loved what your body looked like right now, would it really matter what the number was?

RULES FOR WEIGHING

I have some rules for weighing that I share with my clients and that I think create a healthier relationship with the scale.

The number one rule for weighing yourself is only weigh yourself when you're feeling good. If you're starting an exercise and weight loss program, and you want to track how efficient and effective it is, fine. Get on the scale that one time because you're going to commit to doing something different and to integrating exercise and healthier eating into your life, as a lifestyle change, not as a temporary mechanism for dropping a few pounds.

If you're starting a new program, weigh yourself and then put the scale away for at least eight weeks. Learn to appreciate the results and the progress that you're making by looking in the mirror and being kind to yourself. Pay attention to your body and acknowledge when you notice change or you feel good. Stop discounting small changes and successes because you are focused on the end goal. Instead, replace "but I am not there yet" with ""I'm feeling tighter," or "I'm feeling thinner, and I really feel good." Only then consider weighing yourself . Take your power back and say "I feel good about me today. While I have goals and want to release more weight and look even better, I'm happy, acknowledging and appreciating what has been done so far."

The life you had before is what caused you to get here in the first place. It's not really about the food choices; it's about the emotions underneath those food choices, the real the emotions, which you don't want to experience, feel, or deal with that cause you to overeat or stuff down with food.

While it does feel good to lose weight, it feels better to like your body. I believe you have to like, accept, and take care of your body as it is right now; and all of the motivation that you gain from food, exercise, and self-care should come from a place of love and respect. Next, test your body composition. Visit www.invisiblefitness.com for the online calculator that uses a tape measure to figure out what your body fat percentage is. That's what I use with most of my clients because that way you are forever empowered to measure yourself and there is less need for a trainer. You don't have to have five different people measure you in different places. You, yourself, can track your body fat forever and for free.

When you start to measure the circumference of your neck, chest, waist, hips, thighs, calves and your wrist, be sure to write it all down and keep it. These measurements will help you see progress, and give you specific information about how your body is responding to your exercise program.

The weight on the scale might not change, but maybe you lost three pounds of body fat and three inches along your waist, which would mean you built muscle and lost fat. From there we can understand that your metabolism is now faster than it was when you started. This is all good news when you use all of this information instead of misinterpreting, from the scale alone, that no progress had been made.

Lastly, the rule of weighing is to remind yourself at all times that you are not your weight, and your weight is not a reflection of your self-worth. You are a worthy person, capable of doing anything that you put your mind to, no matter what the number on the scale says. You always have the power to change it, adjust it, and to give yourself some love and compassion. Recognize that you are not your weight and you are not your body-your body responds to your behaviors. Your body is just going to be an indicator of what you're feeling and how you're behaving and that, you can change.

My recommendation is to stop focusing on the weight and heal whatever is eating you up inside. Only then will you free yourself from the need to stuff down uncomfortable emotions with food. Learn to love your body and love yourself where you are right now in order to make lasting, permanent, and healthy changes. Otherwise, you're going to be the hamster on the wheel all the time, giving the power away to the scale.

Let's get started on healing all of this. Release the weight that you're holding on to and shift your body into a place where you love and care for yourself. With that, your body will be happy to change for you because you are loving and respecting it, not shaming it.

LESSONS WILL BE REPEATED UNTIL LEARNED

I remember when I first became a personal trainer and I was living in New York City. It was around the time that the book, **Don't Sweat the Small Stuff** came out. It was all the rage and I remember a highly anxious co-worker of mine finding useful "tips and tricks" in it so he recommended it to me.

Not too long after I purchased my copy, I also heard about **If Life is a Game, These are The Rules** by Dr. Cherie Carter Scott.

She made her first appearance on Oprah and one of my clients recorded the show and gave me my first copy.

While there are gems of wisdom in both, these books represent two different approaches to life that I recognized after reading them. One is about surface level strategy and reaction while the other is about deeper healing and releasing.

As I started out in the fitness industry twenty years ago, my training started with the approach of looking at the outside and how we could make changes that would produce visible results using exercise and diet. I call this the outside-in approach. If you lost weight and felt more energy, it might shift your emotions and beliefs into living life differently.

However, what I have learned is that changing the outside doesn't change the energy inside. To be successful with releasing weight and healing body shame, we have to address the inside-out.

CHAPTER 2

NEW HABITS DON'T FIX THE PROBLEM

"Eventually you will come to understand that love
heals everything, and love is all there is ."

Gary Zukav, the Seat of the Soul

L ET'S SAY YOU'VE TRIED diet after diet, you've done several exercise programs, gone on a retreat, and detox, and they
haven't worked long-term. This is because this is not an external
issue. This is not about misunderstanding *what* to do-it's about
the deeper motivation of the impulse. The root of all of this isn't
physical- it's emotional. Just changing the behavior or swapping
out the behavior for a better habit will not heal the deeper
wound.

Think about a weed again- a very basic concept to understand.
The root is firmly planted in the dirt and as long as that root
is fed by the soil and the water, then it's going to grow again.
Plucking it at the top where you can see it doesn't mean that
that root won't regrow or won't grow into something else. The
weed is your emotional impulse that produces your habit. If you
have only focused on the behavior, the root of the impulse and
emotion is still there, and it's going to show up again.

Sometimes emotions are scary and we don't want to feel them. That is normal but it doesn't mean it's healthy. We think it's normal because everybody is doing it, but it isn't what's going to get you to the greatest depths of happiness and results with both your body and life.

If you're just forcing yourself to repeat the same patterns over and over again such as, joining the gym and eating different foods instead of naturally being inspired from the true depth of who you are with clarity and ease, then it's just clipping the weed off at the top and it's going to grow back. Sometimes the impulse is physical- there are biochemical, neurotransmitter, and hormonal factors that can manifest as an emotional experience. After twenty years of working one on one with clients, I have learned that after we balance the body and gut, we have to heal the heart and soul for lasting success.

I want to share a testimonial of a client who called herself a "lifer"- someone who has been on this weight loss journey for over 20 years and has done many programs.

"I was introduced to JJ Flizanes through a 90 day challenge program to jumpstart my attempt to take control of my health and fitness. The program obviously included directives for eating clean and healthy, and also some recommendations for exercise. I expected all that. In fact, I expected a list of BAD foods that I could never eat again. I expected a brutal exercise regimen that I would need to punish myself with daily.

The program also included a weekly call with JJ. I thought that those calls would be where we would tell how much weight we lost and we would confess if we "cheated" on the diet that week, etc.

Basically, I expected it to be like every other diet or program I had ever joined over the course of my life.

Let's just say that those calls didn't remotely resemble anything I had ever participated in. JJ never asked how much weight I lost. Instead, she wanted to know how I felt. She dug deep into the emotional issues that were causing me to have a constant struggle with my weight. I didn't realize that I had "issues" that were keeping me fat before these meetings.

This was a game changer.

JJ truly deals with the "whole person" to find the root causes of your food issues. She gives you the resources to deal with the issues and helps you make it a daily practice. She never judges. She's not about hitting the number on a scale. Instead, she wants you to be completely in touch with your own body and mind and be able to live a healthy and happy life.

And I did lose 34 pounds in those first 90 days.

I've made changes I can stick to with JJ's program. I now make choices and judge them by "how did that make me feel?" rather than judging my behavior as good or bad. It's a much easier way to deal with food and make the best choices for my body each and every day.

If you want to finally get a little bit uncomfortable and dig deeper to uncover your food issues and then deal with whatever you discover in a healthy way, then you need to talk to JJ!"

Christy H,

WHY SELF LOVE IS IMPORTANT

Everything starts with the relationship you have with yourself-how you talk, look at, present, and feel about yourself.

The most important self-development time in your life is from your birth to about the age of 8 or 9 because it is when you form beliefs from the messages and modeling of other people. These experiences are what create your subconscious mind and act as the foundation of your beliefs. The subconscious mind makes up 88% while your conscious mind, the thoughts you can hear in your head, make up only 12%.

Energetically as well as verbally, through the modeling of your parents, siblings, and other adults that might have lived with you or raised you, the subconscious was formed. Those people made a great impact on your life and their energy was embedded within your cells. Some of the stuff you may come up against on your self-love journey won't even be yours.

A few years ago, at a holiday celebration, there was some conflict that happened at my dinner table between the guests. Hours later, after not being able to sleep, I acknowledged how uncomfortable I was still feeling, and decided to reach out to the therapist I was working with to sort it out. She said, "It sounds like insecurity." I completely identified with that, but I didn't know where it came from.

When I shared it with my husband, he was also perplexed. Insecurity didn't sound like me because I grew up with very supportive parents who still are my biggest cheerleaders but I knew the diagnosis was correct, I just didn't know why or how.

Forty-eight hours later on a vacation with my mother in Jamaica, I noticed the emotions and feelings that was she experiencing while being in a new country, and it was that of insecurity. When she gets nervous, she talks a lot or has very anxious energy and as I watched her, I secretly started to cry.

I didn't tell her I was crying, not because I felt shame, guilt or sadness, it was because now I could see that the insecurity I had been experiencing was hers, not mine.

That energy and way of being was modeled for me, my whole life, and was embedded in me energetically. Think of it as a frequency, tone, or vibration. When you are around a lower frequency, like fear or sadness, it can influence how you are feeling. On the flip side, being around happy, vibrant, positive people can also lift your mood and inspire you.

Now that I understood where it came from, I could use therapeutic tools to heal it. Without the awareness or identification, the patterns keep repeating. If I'm having an experience or a conflict with somebody, and if that conflict keeps repeating itself in my life, I get to choose whether I think that's a random act or if I actually created an opportunity for awareness and healing.

When you dive into self-love practices and look at healing some of these wounds that have been perpetuating in your life, you actually will transform the outcome. Your experience, relationships, feelings, and your body will shift-I promise you.

The journey of self-love takes introspection. It takes care and the same amount of attention you would give a child or someone that you love, because if you can't love and respect yourself, why would you expect someone else to? If you can't stop and give yourself care, love yourself, and ask for what you need, why would somebody swoop in and do it for you?

Doesn't it feel better and stronger to say, "I like myself. I have the amount of self-respect to acknowledge that I'm a good person and I want to take care of myself"? Isn't that what you want to teach your children? Otherwise, you teach (and model) that in order to feel love, other people have to jump through hoops for you. This is called co-dependence and this is an addiction that will perpetuate depression and anxiety.

What we're all searching for is love-it's the end goal, right? Don't you just want to experience and feel happiness and love? If you just dive down underneath all the reasons why you want all the things you want—money, cars, a relationship, a family, a better body—keep going deeper and deeper, what's at the bottom? What is it you really want? You want to feel love and happiness.

What is 100% true is that you can choose to feel that right now. It just has to be a shift of your mindset and interpretation of what's going on. If we always look outside of ourselves to feel love, then it's going to be fleeting, conditional, and based on somebody else's behavior, or our "interpretation" of someone else's behavior. You can't expect other people to change so that you feel good.

I promise that when you can love yourself, you will manifest health and healing that can last, because it's coming from a strong foundation.

The healing doesn't have to be hard, drawn out, and include several years of therapy. I will be providing tools and resources here, in my podcast shows and in The Invisible Fitness Academy so be sure to check out JJFlizanes.com to see what is best to support your journey.

Are you willing to love yourself? Are you willing to also forgive yourself and to heal? Isn't feeling good and having happiness and love what you really want?

CHAPTER 3

SECRET 1: HEAL DIGESTION

―――――――――

"Let food be thy medicine and medicine be thy food ."

Hippocrates

FOOD IS MEDICINE.

As a GREEK-ITALIAN-AMERICAN foodie, my goal is to help you learn to derive pleasures from food and still be able to optimize health. I do not support deprivation or being unsatisfied with your meals. I promise you can learn how to use food in a way that can help you achieve health and well-being, in a way that will taste good!

Digestion is one of the most important functions in our bodies. Basically, the digestive system is designed to turn the food you eat into nutrients, which the body uses for energy, growth, and cell repair. Without eating, we can't survive. Although the concept is simple, the reality is quite complex.

Digestion is an intricate combination of biological interactions and chemical reactions taking place at every stop along the digestive tract, which starts with the mouth, esophagus, stomach, and then continues in the small and large intestine. The gastrointestinal tract is also the largest part of your body's immune system, protecting you against foreign invaders by producing acids and beneficial bacteria that act as a defensive army fighting to protect you from pathogens that find their way inside the body.

A under publicized condition that is rampant and undiagnosed in our society is leaky gut syndrome. Before I explain what it is, here is a list of symptoms that could indicate whether or not you suffer from leaky gut:

» Diagnosis of an autoimmune disease such as celiac, psoriasis, lupus, rheumatoid arthritis, or Hashimoto's

» Diagnosis of chronic fatigue or fibromyalgia

» Skin problems like acne, rosacea, or eczema

» Diagnosis of candida

» Digestive stress such as constipation, gas, bloating, cramps, diarrhea or irritable bowel syndrome (IBS)

» Mood and mind issues such as depression, anxiety, ADD or ADHD

» Hormonal imbalances

» Seasonal allergies or asthma

» Food allergies or food intolerances

Leaky gut is a condition that occurs due to the development of gaps between the cells that make up the membrane that lines your intestinal wall- like tiny tears in the intestines.

These tiny tears allow substances such as undigested food, bacteria, and metabolic waste, which are supposed to be confined to your digestive tract, to escape into your bloodstream. Once you have "torn" the intestinal walls and the integrity of your lining is compromised, there is a flow of toxic substances "leaking out" into your bloodstream -- hence the term leaky gut syndrome.

The body considers this leakage a "foreign substance" sending white blood cells to attack and try to repair the damage, which causes your body to experience significant increases in inflammation. In addition, your immune system may become confused and begin to attack your own body as if it were an enemy, which is autoimmunity.

Often leaky gut syndrome is associated with inflammatory bowel diseases like Crohn's and ulcerative colitis, or celiac disease, but even healthy people can have varying degrees of intestinal permeability leading to a wide variety of health symptoms -- and this is influenced heavily by the foods you choose to eat. Food and toxins associated with causing leaky gut are gluten, dairy, sugar, antibiotics, Motrin, Advil, steroids, acid-reducing drugs, and environmental toxins like mercury, pesticides, and BPA from plastics.

Stress, emotions, and age also contribute to a leaky gut since, emotionally, how we "digest" and process life can have a direct energetic impact on our digesting abilities. If you lack healthy emotional processing and hold onto stress, this will disrupt digestion even with a clean diet. It's common to "get a pit" in your stomach when you are nervous, and this emotional energy will have an impact on how well your body will digest your food. One of the emotional roots of general digestive stress is, "I can't take that in. There are difficulties   with assimilation of experiences and inputs due to generalized dread, repressed rage and/or despairing depression." (Messages from The Body, Michael J Lincoln, Ph.D)

SIGNS OF HEALTHY DIGESTION

Many symptoms of poor digestion are overlooked as if they are "normal". Just because you may always experience gas or bloating doesn't mean normal is healthy or optimal. Elimination and stool are the easiest way to diagnose healthy digestion. For every meal you have, there should be elimination because what goes in also has to come out. One bowel movement a day means you are constipated- this is not healthy digestion. Two to three bowel movements a day that are easy, like soft serve yogurt, are a sign of healthy digestion. If your stool is hard or loose, there is digestive stress. Coffee drinkers would have to give up coffee for a week or more, since coffee is a diuretic and will stimulate elimination, to be able to tell if your body digests well on its own. To learn more and assess your bowel movements, search Bristol Stool Chart.

FOOD ALLERGY VS FOOD SENSITIVITY

Most people think that because they do not have an automatic reaction to a food that it is not a problem. There is a difference between a food allergy and a food intolerance or sensitivity.

A food allergy usually comes on suddenly, happens every time you eat that food and can be life threating. When you're allergic to a substance, your immune system mistakenly believes it is dangerous and produces immunoglobulin E (IgE) antibodies in an attempt to neutralize it. Chemicals such as histamine released into your bloodstream during this process can lead to a battery of symptoms any time you eat the food.

With food sensitivity, your immune system is not involved. Instead, symptoms of food sensitivities may be caused by your body having difficulty breaking down or digesting certain foods or ingredients. Symptoms of food sensitivities usually come on gradually and are not life threatening but can lead to autoimmune disorders and leaky gut.

Research estimates that as much as 60% of the population may have a hidden food sensitivity –particularly to gluten, casein(dairy), soy, wheat, and other common "healthy" foods you enjoy and crave daily.

Food sensitivities and leaky gut cause inflammation, which leads to cell breakdown and damage to DNA. Excessive inflammation also causes damage to your blood vessels. If you don't get the key nutrients and toxins in and out of your cells, you will not release weight efficiently. Instead of counting calories to lose weight, focus on healing your digestion to assist in eliminating any of the above symptoms-weight loss will be a welcomed side effect of healing your gut. Chapter 9 will cover a list of hormones to be tested with your physician, a breakdown of what each is, and how it affects your health. For gut health and inflammation, be sure to consult a physician to measure your C-Reactive Protein (CRP), Insulin, and Homocysteine (A1C) to determine if these are contributing to having a hard time releasing weight.

To start healing your gut, we need to do a combination of removing inflammatory foods and increasing the healthy bacteria to break down any remaining food. The first two foods to remove are gluten and dairy.

WHAT IS GLUTEN?

Gluten is the protein contained in wheat, barley, and rye.

Many people are not able to break down this tough protein; the body perceives this substance as a toxic. Gluten, while in most bread, pastas, crackers, and pastries, can also be hidden. It's in the molds that give chocolate candies their shape and it's also in chewy candies. Food companies and restaurants use it to make soups and gravies thicker, and salad dressings creamier. It keeps dried spices from clumping in their jars. Manufacturers use it to keep candy bars from sticking to the factory conveyor belt. It's in the "caramel coloring" added to soft drinks and in the "natural flavoring," "modified food starch", and "textured vegetable protein" added to thousands of food products. It is used to bind veggie burgers, turkey burgers, and hot dogs. It's even in the decaffeinating process used for coffees and teas and it's a filler in medicines.

In Europe, most physicians check for gluten sensitivity and they find that about one out of every four people are sensitive to gluten. The most effective way to check to see if you are gluten sensitive is a stool test-it's 99.9% accurate. While testing is important, I also encourage you to do an elimination diet to remove this hard to digest protein and allow your body to release inflammation. I will cover how to most easily and effectively do that after we cover dairy and starting you on a high quality probiotic. Be sure to check the resource section for recommended tests for food sensitivities.

WHY DAIRY IS BAD

Dairy is one of the most inflammatory foods in our modern diet, second only to gluten. Like the protein in gluten, the protein in dairy is also hard for humans to digest. Think about it-dairy is the breast milk from cows produced only to fatten calves. Cows, as adults, don't even drink milk. It's also the equivalent of giving human breast milk to an animal. Breast milk from humans is meant for humans. The two components of dairy that tend to cause issues for people are the proteins and the sugar. People who are lactose intolerant don't produce the lactase enzyme, which is required to break down lactose, a sugar found in milk, causing digestive issues whenever they consume dairy products. People who do produce the lactase enzyme but still react poorly to milk are responding to the two proteins found in milk, casein and whey. Casein is a protein with a very similar molecular structure to gluten, and 50% of people who are gluten intolerant are casein intolerant as well.

Milk is also often full of hormones and antibiotics. American dairy farmers have long been injecting cows with a genetically engineered bovine growth hormone called rBGH to increase milk production. This forced increase in milk production often leads to an udder infection in cows called mastitis, which is then treated with courses of antibiotics that can make their way into your dairy products and your body. It's suspected that this is one of the reasons young girls are starting the menstrual cycle earlier in life and why more women and men have hormonal imbalances. If you are concerned about calcium, you can get food based, non-dairy calcium from sources such as almonds, tofu, collard greens, broccoli, kale, okra, bok choy, edamame, figs, oranges, sardines, canned salmon, and white beans. We don't need to consume dairy.

START TAKING PROBIOTICS

What is a probiotic? Live microorganisms that are found anywhere from your mouth to your anus-the entire tube actually has microorganisms that can benefit your health. We call them probiotics, which means "for life" in Greek. They are friendly bacteria that help to support your body in so many ways. Probiotics aid the body in breaking down nutrients in the right molecular size so your immune system doesn't overreact or underreact.

There's certain kinds of microbes that actually keep bad bacteria in your intestinal lining and can extract more calories from food so these microbes improve the way that your body metabolizes your calories. Probiotics are one of the things that can help improve how you get nutrients from your gut into your bloodstream.

We're often craving sugar when we are actually craving nutrients. Beneficial bacteria in your gut can help you feel more at home in your body, more relaxed, and improve your ability to eat in a way that's geared more towards what your body needs.

A few recent studies gave two groups of rats a low-calorie diet- both groups were receiving the same amount of calories. However, in one group, they added a probiotic into the food. What they found was that the group that had the probiotic lost about 30% more weight than the group of rats that were consuming just the food alone. Leading researchers are now starting to look at the power of adding either cultured or fermented foods that contain probiotics or adding in a supplement probiotic in a weight loss program.

YOUR GUT IS YOUR SECOND BRAIN

About 75% to maybe even 90% of your immune system lives in your gut. Which is also where you produce a lot of your neurotransmitter brain type chemicals like serotonin. Probiotics can help you experience better moods as well as health because they help with proper digestion and elimination.

Foods that typically are naturally rich in these probiotics help improve and stimulate peristalsis and the muscular rhythms that you need to move food through your large intestine and into the colon. While we think that we need to get many of our vitamins from pills, actually, these probiotics can produce vitamin K as well as some of the B vitamins that we desperately need. Probiotics help us absorb minerals, eliminate toxins, and enhance our nutritional status just by making sure that we're getting a good dose of them on a regular basis.

If you take a look around the world, we didn't even have probiotics on shelves 30 years ago because we were getting them in our cultured foods like yogurt and sauerkraut. Originally, how people got some of their probiotics was through these cultured foods, which all cultures around the world have learned how to do, mostly to enhance how long the food could sit on the shelf.

Prior to refrigeration, not long ago, people kept their milk, butter, and yogurts in a cool cellar. Yogurt could stay in a cool cellar at around 40 degrees for one month before it went bad. That's why it was such a popular thing for people to culture foods; you could keep vegetables, dairy products, and even fish a lot longer if you had them cultured because it's a natural preservative.

Enjoy cultured foods like kimchi, a national Korean dish made up of fermented cabbage and seasonings, raw sauerkraut, as they do in Germany or like in the Balkan and Russian countries that use beets and make beet kvass; they culture beets because it's food that grows so easily up in those very cold regions. Eating cultured foods would be the ideal way to get them, but not everybody likes that strong kind of cultured, sour taste.

PREBIOTICS

You can help your body make more probiotics naturally by consuming prebiotics. Prebiotics act as food for probiotics. In other words, probiotics eat prebiotics. Prebiotic foods are fibers called inulins and fructooligosaccharides. These particular fibers actually stimulate the growth of some of your own good guys, like the good flora. A good example of some of these fibers would be a banana, artichokes, and sunchokes. You can also get prebiotics from raw and cooked onions, raw garlic, raw leeks, raw dandelion greens, raw asparagus, and raw chickory root; these foods are going to help feed, or give the food source to grow more bifidobacteria and acidophilus, which are probiotics that just naturally occur in the human GI tract. To start growing your own probiotics, consume a minimum amount of a quarter of a cup. There's no downside to having more, but you're going to want at least enough so that you're going to be able to give those bacteria something to grow on.

ANTIBIOTICS

Antibiotics wipe out many of the good bacteria but also all the bad bacteria. Without adding probiotics back into your gut, the bad bacteria will start to rush in because everyone is looking for real estate along your GI tract. If you have been on antibiotics for any length of time, your gut is starting from scratch. You should immediately take a high-quality probiotic supplement to avoid a buildup of yeast, which is one of the first things that start to come out because yeast will break down the carnage from all of those cells that just died. Somebody has to clean up all those bacteria cells, and the garbage man is yeast. That's why people will frequently get a yeast infection right after they've been on antibiotics. In fact, if you're on an antibiotic, you should make sure that you're taking your probiotic three hours after. If you take your antibiotic first thing in the morning, then take a probiotic or eat some cultured foods before you go to bed or somewhere during the day to help get some of the more effective bacterial strains back into your body.

WHICH PROBIOTICS?

The human genome project has been discovering that there are certain bacterial strains that are outstanding and each have different jobs. For example, if a woman has yeast infections, there are certain strains of probiotics that are specific for the vaginal cavity and uterus, because they live in that area. If you have excessive dental problems, there is probiotic toothpaste. We can get very specific but at the same time generalize what strains are critical for most conditions.

One of the biggest bacterial species that we know have been effective is Lactobacillus acidophilus. It is a very effective strain of beneficial bacteria that works to help improve your immune system. Bifidobacteria, another super strain, is one that children get when they start suckling from their mother. Therefore, we've developed a relationship with these kinds of bacteria that really help improve the immune system components in the body.

We have acid in our stomach that's so strong that many of these probiotics are killed right there and they never make it down to the lower gut. Pay the little extra money to make sure it's acid- and bile-resistant, so that it actually survives through the first stage of digestion, which is getting past the stomach. Visit invisiblefitness.com for brands and products I use and recommend.

CHAPTER 4

ELIMINATION DIETS

———

"You don't know what you've got, til it's gone ."

Tom Keifer, lead singer of Cinderella

NOW THAT YOU UNDERSTAND the top two inflammatory foods, an elimination diet can further help identify obstacles to releasing weight. Elimination diets are used to identify food sensitivities, which are cumulative, compounding, and can create leaky gut. You may not have an obvious reaction within a few days, which is why it is important to allow 2-4 weeks for your body to adjust.

Before my wedding, I wanted to do some kind of detox program. From growing up with mercury fillings in my teeth, I tested high for mercury in my tissues. I chose a heavy metal detox because high levels of mercury can lead to Alzheimer's and other degenerative diseases. Long story short, I sent away for this mercury detox and gave myself two months to do it before the wedding, in case my skin broke out or something unexpected happened.

Maybe it was because of where I was living, someone maybe stole it or there was a problem with the mail, but it never came.

Now, I was a month away from the wedding and wanted to replace that detox with something less risky on my skin. Gluten sensitivity and the negative effects from gluten were becoming more popular, so I thought, "Well, why not try that?"

With nothing to lose, I did what I needed to do to prepare. Within the next 10 days I lost six pounds- of water, not six pounds of fat. Every month around my cycle, I would have what I considered was menstrual bloating. I just thought, "Well, I'm bloated, so that's part of what happens when it's this time of the month." What I realized is that, no, that's not what happens; that's what happens when I eat gluten. It was a real eye-opener for me, and so gluten was the first thing I eliminated out of my diet. My mother followed and while her weight loss wasn't as fast, she lost seven or eight pounds over two or three months.

STEPS OF AN ELIMINATION DIET

Once you have overcome the resistance to the idea of eliminating a food group from your diet for 2-4 weeks, it is very important to follow these steps to ensure the best experience and results. If you feel restricted, you're not going to do it because the thought brings up fear and discomfort about, "What am I going to eat?" I've been there-I understand.

For most of my life, I was a cheese-aholic. Giving up gluten was easy because there were several ways to replace the foods I might crave. However, I craved cheese so much that the thought of not having it created a lot of resistance. It took a couple of years of me getting tired of blowing my nose, and knowing full-well that it was coming from dairy, to try eliminating dairy because I ate a lot of cheese.

First, identify your symptoms and the correlating food that may be causing it. Dairy is usually the culprit for when you're blowing your nose, have a lot of mucus or drainage, phlegm or constipation. Eczema is also usually dairy, as well as other skin conditions. Another important clue is that the food you crave the most is usually the food your body has a hard time digesting. Decide if you want to eliminate one food at a time or more. If you are looking for faster release of weight, I'd suggest giving up gluten and dairy at the same time. However, this will be more challenging if these are still a large part of your diet, so make sure to complete the second step very thoroughly.

Secondly, make a list of your comfort foods and go-to snacks, and then replace them with a dairy-free and/or gluten-free option. A great idea if you want to take it a step further would be to make a list of what you normally eat, just in general. What are your normal three breakfast, lunch, dinner, dessert and/or snack choices? Point by point, find a replacement so you can keep your "habits" the same, we are just going to change the ingredients. Make sure to read all labels, as there are hidden sources of gluten and dairy in many products.

We forget what's in our food because we identify dairy as milk. Therefore, if you're not drinking milk, you may think, "Well, I don't drink milk." However, you may have cheese, cream in your coffee, ice cream, sour cream, cream cheese, or yogurt. Look at the ingredients that are in the foods that you're eating, not just the food itself. The only "dairy" that can stay in your diet is organic, grass fed butter because butter is all fat, there is no protein or whey in butter, and most people can digest it so don't be so quick to give up good quality, organic, grass fed, hormone free butter.

To make it easier, I have set up a place on ***theinvisiblefitness.com*** where you can purchase many of my favorite choices. You can also download a list of my recommended name brand products that are gluten and dairy free, to take out some of the guesswork. Finding the products that taste the best to you is part of the initial work, but once you find them, it makes life and eating much easier.

In 2008, when I first went gluten free, there were not a lot of choices on the market. One brand of gluten free bread felt like a brick so it was a turn off for eating bread. The allergy free food market has exploded over the last 10 years so there are many choices out there to sift through. If you try something you do not like, ask for recommendation for something better. I am positive we can find you something you will not only tolerate, but also truly enjoy.

Now that you've gone to the store and purchased the gluten free and dairy free items, try them and make sure you like them. Within your calendar, pick 2-4 weeks that don't have too many parties, birthdays, or celebrations, where there is going to be a limited menu that may cause feelings of restriction. In the case of the unexpected celebration, instead of focusing on what you can't have, ask yourself "what can I have". Bringing food to share or eating beforehand are also options to help you stay true to this experiment.

July 1st, 2008 was the first day I became gluten free and to this day, I may have gluten 3-5 times a year for very special occasions and for foods that I cannot get or make gluten free, like certain Greek Foods. Although this past Christmas, I did make a gluten free pastry dough for a Spanakopita because I had no desire to eat the traditional gluten filled dough. While it didn't act the same, (instead of being fluffy, it was crunchy) my husband and I really enjoyed them.

I went mostly dairy free in 2010, when I had reached my tolerance limit of nose blowing at night and to this day, I have dairy once or twice a month. If I am sharing a gluten free pizza with friends who don't want the dairy free cheese, I make sure that I have taken my probiotics and add some digestive enzymes to help me break down the cheese and minimize the side effects.

Around 2013, I became Paleo, which is grain free as well as gluten and dairy free. Just like the commitment needed to stay gluten free and then dairy free, Paleo was a choice I made when I was ready. When you learn how to replace foods you love with healthier, low inflammatory choices, it's easier to clean up your diet and stick to it because there are no feelings of restriction.

A side benefit of a low carb, low inflammatory diet is that cravings are reduced or even eliminated. Before going gluten free, I would salivate at the smell of pizza, if I were hungry or not. After one month of being gluten free, I drove past a pizza place smelling the pizza and my mouth stayed dry. That was when I really understood the biochemical response that inflammatory food had on the body.

I have long time clients that I work with in Arizona and once a year I cook them a Paleo meal to show them that they can eat delicious food and not miss grains, gluten, or dairy. Year after year, I get rave reviews for the food, most of which have been featured on the Fit 2 Love Podcast show and The Easy Paleo, Gluten & Dairy Free Cooking show that I have on iTunes as well as *jjflizanes.tv.*

Here's the thing, you can't be sure, until you try it. I was skeptical of wheat causing problems in the body for 10 years. The first time I heard about it, I thought that was ridiculous because I didn't think I had any symptoms. Then I tried it, released six pounds, reduced food cravings, and even had more energy.

One caution to watch out for on elimination diets is overeating "gluten free" carbohydrates. Two years after I went gluten-free, I lead a group of women through a gluten-free elimination diet. They replaced gluten with gluten free versions of all their fun foods, cookies, breads, pastas, cakes, and gained weight because they were eating more sugar, starch, and calories. Start by only replacing the things that you normally eat. An elimination diet is not a green light to overeat new things that are full of starch and sugar, because that can cause weight gain.

At the end of the elimination diet, add one food back in and see how you respond to it. Dairy will cause more immediate symptoms, so remember that effects from gluten can be cumulative and show up later in the form of digestive stress or an autoimmune disorder.

If this is your first elimination diet, do it as an experiment. It may take some time, mentally and emotionally, to decide whether or not to live this way, so be patient with yourself – you have to be ready. Remember, I love food; I am Greek and Italian so trust me when I tell you that if I can do this, you can do this. Make it fun. Make it exploratory. It's only 2-4 weeks, and this can be a fun experiment that could even be a life-changing experience. As you prepare for the elimination diet, we have to address the carbohydrate and sugar issue.

CHAPTER 5

UNDERSTANDING SUGAR

"Up to 40% of US healthcare expenditures are for
diseases directly related to the overconsumption
of sugar ."

Credit Suisse research Institute's 2013 study

S UGAR, IS ONE OF THE MOST misunderstood foods in our diet.
From sugar free substitutes to low glycemic versions of
sweeteners, what the body does with sugar is a big reason why
people find it hard to lose weight, and keep it off. It is also one
of the biggest contributors to many health issues but it is often
overlooked because it's "food". From chronic pain, diabetes,
obesity, high blood pressure, mood swings, headaches, anxiety,
and brain fog, the misunderstanding of what sugar is may be
keeping us sick and fat.

First, all carbohydrates turn into sugar. The only thing that
maybe varies is just how quickly they turn to sugar. Whether
you're looking at an apple, apple juice, soda, or a piece of bread,
they all eventually turn to sugar.

The body will break down foods that contain carbohydrates
into sugar, and then uses something called insulin, which is like

a carrier to help transport that sugar from your bloodstream into the muscles where then the body can store them. Using the liver as an example, imagine the muscles in the liver are like a sponge, the body will continue to fill up the holes in the muscles of your liver until it reaches a saturation point. After that point, anything more that you consume, your body has to store it. That's when it starts storing some of that sugar in the form of fat in the liver. A major health crisis we have right now is actually fatty liver.

The second thing is the excess amount of carbs that the average person consumes that will to turn to fat and usually goes into the belly, because that's a quick and easy way to store it. Anybody that has belly fat is probably eating more carbohydrates than their body is able to utilize for energy.

If you are eating too many carbs and sending all this sugar into your body, you are also increasing insulin production. We now recognize insulin as a hormone that contributes to fast aging. Insulin is great, in terms of getting sugar into your cells where your body needs it, but if you start putting too much insulin out, it actually has the ability to drive more fat into your fat cells.

Excess insulin contributes to things like blood pressure problems, heart palpitations, and shrinking your brain. There are also mood swings from the ups and downs of having too much sugar in your blood. That up and down rollercoaster effect can really increase anxiety and mood swings, general fatigue and even infections.

One of the first things that happens when you overload your body with sugar is the immune system gets overwhelmed. The immunity is the key response team, like your inner paramedics, fire department, and police department that's looking to respond to emergencies. When you start pumping too much sugar into your bloodstream, it becomes difficult for the immune system to work effectively.

If you've ever dropped sugar on the floor and something wet was already there, it gets sticky. Well, the same thing is true in your blood. If you have too much sugar in your blood and you don't clear all of it out, it ends up sticking to the red blood cells of your body, so blood cells will start to clump together.

If they clump together, then they can't get into the tiny little capillaries that feed your eyes, fingertips, and toes. One of the first signs of pre-diabetes is that eyesight isn't as good because they're not getting the blood flowing in and out of those tiny little capillaries, or their fingertips or their toes have lost circulation. These little tiny capillaries are not receiving this oxygenated blood because they're clumped and preventing one blood cell going into one capillary at a time. These are all signs of early diabetes, but there's a lot more. Anytime you have excess sugar, you're going to have excess insulin. Insulin is the carrier, and insulin makes your cells more brittle and blood vessels a little bit less elastic.

SUGAR BREAKDOWN

How quickly sugar breaks down is related to the amount of fiber. An apple is going to take longer to break down than drinking a glass of apple juice because there's more fiber in it. One of the reasons why it is important to get plenty of fiber in your diet is that foods higher in fiber are going to slow down that sugar in the bloodstream. Eat fruit instead of drinking fruit juice-an apple has less sugar than a glass of apple juice.

It takes three apples to make an 8-ounce glass of apple juice. Drinking apple juice will take five minutes but it could take hours to eat three apples. Most people wouldn't even finish three apples unless they were super hungry. Chewing slowly slows down that sugar entering into the bloodstream, which helps reduce the amount of insulin needed and the body can really handle it better. For health and weight loss reasons, moderately active people want to focus on getting 100 grams or less of carbohydrates daily. Rather than counting calories, focus on monitoring your daily intake of carbohydrates and sugar.

SWEETENER LESSON 101

Avoid artificial sweeteners because they can actually raise your insulin levels. Artificial sweeteners vary in their sweetness capacity, anywhere from 10 times sweeter than sugar up to 400 times sweeter than sugar. When you put something on your tongue that's 400 times sweeter than sugar, this immediately stimulates your pancreas to say, "Uh-oh. Something sweet is coming. Let's start putting out insulin." Even though you're not putting calories in, like with a diet soda, insulin is something that has its own impact on your health.

The second thing is that when those artificial sweeteners go into the gut, we have certain types of bacteria that will extract more calories from the foods that you consume, particularly around artificial sweeteners. The artificial sweeteners communicate to that group of bacteria, like flipping a switch, to extract more calories. Even though you may be consuming something that has one or two calories, like a diet soda, this type of bacteria is able to extract more calories from the other foods that you're consuming. This is something that was surprising as researchers started looking more into artificial sweeteners.

The last thing is that they change your taste buds. The taste buds start to shift to crave things that are sweeter than we would normally crave and this has an impact even on your endocrinology and metabolism. Diet soda is worse than regular soda, and can cause weight gain for the reasons that they steal the increase of insulin from the pancreas and change our gut bacteria causing an increased craving for sweet.

You really have to be a good label reader because there are so many drinks and beverages on the market right now that have become more aware of the fact that consumers are trying to cut back on artificial sweeteners. Sometimes what they're doing is using some artificial sweeteners along with stevia.

We have to talk about agave because everybody thinks agave is like the darling and we should be using it because it comes from the agave plant, but it also is super high in fructose. A good way of explaining fructose is it's almost like supercharged kindling. When fructose breaks down, it tends to put out a lot of heat in the body. The agave that's being manufactured right now is like a super condensed fructose syrup. It doesn't really have much nutrient value. You'd be better off to switch to using a little bit of honey. Agave is like 70% to 90% high fructose corn syrup or more of a super condensed fructose syrup.

APPROVED SUGAR SUBSTITUTES

The first is stevia, an all-natural, no calorie sweetener that comes from a plant. The flowers produce a very sweet, but slightly bitter tasting flower. Processing the flower and leaves creates a sweetener that's about 30 times sweeter than sugar.

Not nearly the intensely sweet that you get with aspartame or sucralose, but it's still sweet.

Stevia is very safe and can be used to sweeten most dishes and drinks, but the challenge with stevia is sometimes you get a little bit of a bitter taste. Food manufacturers as well as drink and beverage companies have been challenged with this bitter taste because many of them are interested in trying to sweeten foods in a more natural way. Some drink companies are using just small amounts of it with the sucralose or regular sugar to find the right blend. Stevia can be a good alternative just be aware of the fact that because of it being bitter, it won't be the best choice for every food and beverage substitute- all stevia products and brands vary in taste as well.

The next best sugar substitute is Luo Han, which is found in China and is a bit more expensive than stevia. It's about two calories in a teaspoon while white table sugar is four. It's a fruit that's been used as a sweetener for centuries, and is about 200 times sweeter than sugar. The good news is that the FDA added it to the Generally Recognized as Safe (or GRAS) list in 2009. It goes into the bloodstream a little bit slower and is not something that's going to raise blood sugars as quickly. However, it's still 200 times sweeter than sugar, so you still have some of those other issues such as your taste threshold is going to be altered by it. Nevertheless, it certainly has the safe status that many of the other artificial sweeteners do not and have not made that list.

Another safe sugar substitute is xylitol. One of the key things that is nice about xylitol is that it's a sugar alcohol. Anything with "-ol" at the end of the name means that it has the sweetness of sugar, but it kind of functions in the body a little bit more like alcohol so it contains fewer calories. Xylitol, in particular, improves the bacteria that live in your mouth. That's why many chewing gum manufacturers will use xylitol because it actually improves the overall bacterial. You can also find it in some toothpaste or mouthwashes.

The downside with xylitol is that it can produce loose stool because the alcohols aren't digested very effectively towards the end of the digestive process. Some people might notice that they have a little bit of thin stools, but xylitol, in comparison, has a great effect on your blood sugar, so it's a much better choice than using plain old sugar.

Coconut and date sugars are lower glycemic and less processed but they are still sugar. Honey has medicinal and immune system properties but will still spike insulin so use sparingly. High-quality unprocessed honey contains natural antioxidants, enzymes, amino acids, vitamins, and minerals. Unfortunately, most of the honey has been treated with an excessive heating process that can destroy some of the critical natural enzymes, vitamins, and minerals. Choose a high grade, less processed and filtered honey.

CHAPTER 6

WHY PALEO

"Your original 'factory setting' is to be an efficient fat-burning beast!"

Mark Sisson, the primal Blueprint

THE PALEO DIET IS A grain and legume free diet, which will translate into lower glycemic because it is less sugar. We are Paleolithic people in the sense that our genetics have only changed .02 percent in the four million years we have been on the planet. Our genetics and all of our systems, GI tract, teeth, enzymes, and every aspect of every cell membrane is designed to eat a Paleolithic diet.

The Paleolithic diet is the hunter gather diet-what cavemen ate. A very high portion of their diet was related to good healthy protein from animals, fish, and birds that were free range and grass fed. They also ate whatever nuts, berries, roots, wild vegetables, or any of those kinds of foods that they could gather. They didn't have pesticides, hormones, and antibiotics in the food that they were gathering and the wild meat and fish were not corn fed- they didn't even have corn!

The macronutrients that kept that body fat low and muscle mass high was divided into around 30% protein from lean sources,

30% from very healthy fats, and then about 30-40% from more high fiber, unrefined carbohydrates in the form of vegetables. The Paleolithic diet included about a hundred grams of fiber a day from vegetables, roots, and berries where our SAD diet, the Standard American Diet, has one-tenth the amount of fiber that we need to move waste through our bodies. Fiber is extremely important to help you maintain a good weight. However, the recommendation from the American Dietary Association is still only 25 grams when the preventive care physicians are recommending 40 or 50 grams. Dairy, beans, and legumes have come around in the last ten thousand or so years and we're really not designed to digest and assimilate those foods.

WHY I AM NOT VEGAN

Most people hear the term "Vegan" and automatically think that this is the healthiest diet out there because there are no animal products, but many people on a Vegan diet gain weight and suffer certain side effects of not having all the nutrients their body needs. Because of the focus on meat free food, Vegans tend to eat too many starchy carbohydrates which then breakdown into sugar in the body.

Let me start with a few disclaimers. First, if you are vegan, well educated, and aware of the nutrients that your body needs, I am not trying to change you. I respect the choice not to eat animals, when your beliefs create an emotional concern for the planet. I'd love to support every Vegan to do the best job possible in eating to support your body and beliefs.

Second, this chapter is about biochemistry and genetics. If you are on a Vegan diet or aspire to be, I will outline the common mistakes and help you prepare your meals and optimize your health. A Vegan diet is a plant based diet that excludes all animal products but I promote a Paleo diet, which does include animal products, however, like a Vegan diet, should aim to be rich in vegetables and colors. Whether you're Paleo or Vegan, it is important to be consuming more vegetables and high-quality fats.

FOOD MYTH #1: MEAT IS UNHEALTHY

Not all meat is created equal. Feedlot beef, which is what you find in most grocery stores, tend to raise cholesterol. In the Paleo camp, there is this distinction of grass-fed meats and lamb. Grass-fed meat is significantly different in its nutrition profile. There's a lot more omega-3's, Vitamin A, and Vitamin D- more benefits because there's a lot more nutrients. Animals that have the opportunity to spend a good part of their life eating grasses, like in wild game or even just free-range animals are going to have the ability to transform the minerals that are found in those grasses into their tissues in comparison to feedlot animals.

The Paleo Diet is trying to embrace the foods that go back to what our hunter-gatherer ancestors were eating- it was much more wild game. If you're eating industrial factory-farmed animals, you are definitely going to defeat the purpose of going Paleo. Seek out grass-fed, antibiotic and hormone-free poultry and meats.

WHY EAT MEAT?

Animals concentrate nutrition. Most of us are being shortchanged on trace minerals in our daily diets. Grasses, or any kind of plant foods, offer tremendous amount of minerals when consuming 8 to 12 pounds of it a day, which a cow easily can do. This will give you higher levels of zinc, magnesium, manganese, and iron, for example. There are other minerals that would be greater in meat that would require a Vegan to consume large amounts of plant food, which is a challenge that many Vegans have through chewing food. If you include juicing, they might be able to do so. However, if you're just chewing, you're going to feel like a cow all day. You're going to have to be consuming 8-12 pounds of vegetables in order to be able to get that mineral-rich diet that naturally you can get in animal foods.

FOOD MYTH #2: CHOLESTEROL IS BAD

Cholesterol is a wonderful hormone and widely misunderstood. In the late 70's and 80's, a researcher named Ancel Keys looked at the connection between our cholesterol levels and saturated fats in the blood. Some of this research indicated that eggs had 250 milligrams of cholesterol. The food industry then really came down on eggs, but it really wasn't the egg that caused the problem-it was the toast, jam and the sugar. It was the foods that elevated blood sugar levels that had the most to do with raising cholesterol unnaturally, but at the time, people couldn't see the connection between carbohydrates and grains, and the impact that it has on cholesterol levels. Now we see it, but it can take 10 to 12 years to get a new idea embedded into people's way of thinking, and then it's really hard to get it out.

Cholesterol is a necessary hormone that is a precursor to many things such as Vitamin D and Co-enzyme Q10. Cholesterol also makes your pregnenolone, which is a master "mother" hormone. We need adequate amounts of pregnenolone in order to be able to make other hormones like testosterone, estrogen, and progesterone, naturally. Even cortisol and DHEA, the adrenal hormones, come directly from pregnenolone. Foods like egg yolks, that contain cholesterol, also contain choline, which creates phosphatidylcholine- one of the key connecting points in the brain neurons. It has a calming impact on our brain chemistry as well as on our hormonal chemistry. Regular cholesterol, that is not inflamed or oxidized, is not bad cholesterol. A Vegan diet that contains no animal products will be lacking in cholesterol and can affect your brain chemistry and natural hormone production.

It's the oxidized low-density lipoprotein (LDL) that damages blood vessels and creates plaque. If you have inflammation contributing to that process, you're on your way to chronic degenerative disease. Reduce excessive inflammation in your body by eliminating gluten, dairy, and sugar. Include good anti-oxidants and anti-inflammatory compounds such as Resveratrol (found in red wine), and spices like Turmeric (Curcumin).

HOW MUCH PROTEIN

For optimal energy, nutrients, and fat burning, our diets want to get close to 30-30-40; 30% lean, wild protein, 30% healthy fats and up to 40% carbohydrates and fiber coming mostly from plants. The general rule is half of your ideal body weight in grams of protein a day. A 130lb woman would want to aim for 65-70 grams of protein a day unless engaging in more intense resistance training or long durance sports.

Vegetable do have protein but to get 30% of your diet in protein, a Vegan would have to be constantly consuming all day to reach that number. Let's take a serving of broccoli, a half a cup cooked, is about 1.5 grams of protein. There is protein in there, but that's not going to be enough. Maybe you increase the serving to two cups of broccoli, which is probably what most people could consume without getting too full or sick of it. You'd be getting about maybe four, maybe six grams of protein at the most which is not going to give you a sufficient amount unless you're adding some beans, grains, nuts or seeds.

If we compare a handful of meat, chicken, or eggs, there are 14 grams of protein in two eggs, which is very efficient to getting closer to that range of 65 or 70 grams. If you are getting your protein with beans and grains, you'll be eating many starchy calories, which are then going to convert into sugar and probably stored as body fat. You will be getting more calories than you actually need.

WHAT ABOUT SOY?

Soy falls into a category of legumes, which are beans and lentils. One of the things that we know about soybeans is that, first of all, about 80%-90% of all the soy that's being grown right now is not organic and it may be genetically modified. It's one of the more popular commodity foods that are being used to help feed and fatten pigs, cattle, or chickens. Unless you're somebody who's going to properly prepare the anti-nutrients that are found in soy (by the way, all legumes need to be properly prepared), you are probably putting yourself at risk for some thyroid issues. There's an affinity between soy and thyroid concerns.

Soy that's been properly prepared has been inoculated with some bacteria, like in the case of miso, miso soup, or tempeh.

Tempeh is an Indonesian food in which has added probiotics to help break down those soybeans so that they're more digestible. They don't have many of the anti-nutrients that make it difficult to absorb, and they have less affinity for the thyroid gland. So that's a biggie for Vegans to be aware of, that organic soy is one way that you're going to keep the GMOs out, but then the second thing is to look at soy and make sure that you're using soy that's fermented.

Soy protein isolate is a very common ingredient that's used in hundreds of products like bars-it's so cheap. Processed soy foods become excitotoxins, and they have a negative brain impact and cause cellular degeneration. Excitotoxins speed up brain processes and make people feel hyperactive or agitated. Dr. Russell Blaylock wrote the book **Excitotoxins: The Taste That Kills**. It's a great book to look up if you consume soy or want to learn more. There is a huge growth area in the marketplace right now for plant-based proteins, which are using a pea and rice combination. Vega, Arbonne, and Sun Warrior are three of my favorite Vegan, soy free proteins and you can get 18 to 20 grams of protein in a scoop. This is a good way to supplement a Vegan diet, without adding more starchy carbs and excess calories.

WHAT ABOUT JUICING?

As we have already discussed, when you are Paleo, you can get many minerals from eating meat because of massive amount of grasses that the animals consume. However, if you are not eating good quality, grass fed meat, you might be lacking in nutrients and minerals the same as non-meat eaters who are not supplementing them back into the body. Juicing may be high in sugar and low in fiber but it is one of the best ways to get in large doses of mineral and nutrients. Dr. Russell Blaylock, an oncologic neurosurgeon out of the University of Mississippi, promotes the whole idea of nutrition being important for preventing cancer. Anything you do that helps prevent cancer is also going to help prevent cardiovascular disease, metabolic syndrome, diabetes, hypertension, and high cholesterol. His number one recommendation is to get twelve servings of vegetables and fruits a day. Now, most of us won't chew that many in a day but we can drink it through extraction, blending or making vegetables soups. Vegetables are also alkaline and will help balance and neutralize acid from all animal products, stress, toxins, and medications. Blending is great to get the fiber included but if you find you do not like the taste, try juicing instead. Start with whichever tastes best and is easiest to do often. There are a few recipes for both on the Fit 2 Love Podcast Show, *jjflizanes.tv* and Easy, Paleo, Gluten & Dairy Free Cooking show on iTunes.

CHAPTER 7

SECRET 2: GET SMART EXERCISE

"Lack of activity destroys the good condition of every human being, while movement and methodical physical exercise save it and preserve it ."

Plato

A S A PERSONAL TRAINER for twenty years, I can say that this is a topic I am extremely passionate about. It's a topic that I think deserves more respect than it gets in the medical industry because smart exercise includes working with many sciences: anatomy, physiology, physics, and biomechanics, to start.

What is **Smart Exercise**? If you are going to spend time exercising, make it count! Smart exercise is focused, carefully structured exercise that is safe for your joints, effective in building muscle or burning calories, includes a neurological component of control, muscle activation, and is well-rounded to work all muscles over time and increase balance.

As a good financial planner would do, you create your exercise based on the end in mind while considering the current fitness level and environment. For several years, I had branded myself an Exercise Architect because creating a safe and effective plan for someone entails knowing how their unique structure works, and working with that structure to honor its abilities and limitations.

During my first personal training certification, one of my instructors got up in the front of the room and said in a very loud voice, "I have 11 injuries, don't do what I did!"

That was all I needed to hear to understand that the choices you make about your exercise, will affect your joints in the future, either near or far. Mind you, this instructor was an ex Mr. Olympian so the likelihood that many of us would be training like him was slim but the point remained that you can build muscle and preserve your joints, or you could build muscle and wreck your joints.

The problem has been that most people don't want to talk or think about joints until there is already pain or injury. At 25 years old, I was talking about joint integrity to perspective clients and no one cared- they wanted weight loss. Because I focus on helping to prevent injury, I attracted many clients with several injuries because the average personal trainer didn't have the science background to work them out safely.

Let's assume everyone wants weight loss, all my recommendations will be made with that as the #2 focus, second only to making sure your exercise doesn't injure you because that will derail your weight loss efforts.

If you do high intensity, uncontrolled movements to burn calories but put your joints at risk, you may lose weight temporarily but when you inevitably have joint pain and it becomes irritating to exercise, you will lose those results in time.

WHAT IS METABOLISM?

Your metabolism is the rate at which you burn calories at rest. I often refer to it as your gas tank- how much gas does your tank need? There are two main factors, besides hormones, that contribute to what creates this number. First is your nervous system. Next is the amount of active tissue you have-aka muscle.

Let's start by focusing on the nervous system. Imagine a Type A person who is go-go-go all day long. Someone who talks, thinks, and moves fast. This person is burning "extra" calories by their high intensity energy output.

Then there's the Type B person who is real chill and sort of lays around, the couch potato or the person you can barely get off the couch to go take a walk around the block- think surfer dude. That person probably has a slower metabolism in terms of nervous system.

The foundation of your nervous system is part of who you are and, in my opinion, should be left alone. Many people try fat-burning pills, which act like speed for your nervous system and have many negative side effects such as severe mood swings, heart palpitations, restlessness, elevated cardiac stress, and even death. Fat burning pills will work to burn calories, which is why they are still on the market, but the risk will outweigh the benefit-please avoid them.

The second factor of metabolism is your active tissue or muscle- this is what I want to focus on. Muscle moves bone and the stronger your muscles are, the easier it is to move. The more you focus on building and sustaining muscle, the more you can

avoid common injuries that occur due to aging. Building and maintaining muscle also helps preserve bone density, aids with balance, natural hormone production, and improves memory and brain function, which can prevent Alzheimer's disease.

The easiest tool that gives the most amount of relevant information is to measure your body composition. At home methods will focus on your body fat, and not tell you how much muscle you have. Fat is inactive and requires no energy (calories), which is why I recommend that people focus on decreasing your body fat instead of getting on the scale.

Machines used by medical and fitness professionals can often tell you how many pounds of lean mass (muscle) you have as well as the intra cellular and extra cellular water you are carrying. The water readings indicate the health of your cell walls and their ability to transport nutrients inside the cell. It's a good reading to have done, especially if you have health concerns, but it's not crucial at this point for general weight loss.

Adding more active tissue will increase the number of calories you need each day, and therefore, increase your metabolism naturally. If you create your program to focus on building muscle and reducing body fat, you are guaranteed to look and feel successful without even needing to get on a scale. There is probably no other subject that generates more emotional resistance and limiting beliefs, that stop you before you start, than exercise.

MYTH #1: LIFTING WEIGHTS WILL MAKE ME BULKY

This myth stops women especially from burning fat and increasing their metabolism. The fear that lifting weights will make you look like a body builder can't be further from the truth! First, whether they are on enhancers or not, most competitive body builders spend hours and hours at the gym every day.

Actually, I would never recommend that for anyone since bodybuilding is the same addiction as anorexia in reverse (more on that in Chapter 12).

Many bodybuilders are on steroids, creatine, or HGH (Human Growth Hormone). They're on a supplement to enhance their ability to build muscle and they're retaining more water. When thinking about resistance training, and it's not just "weights", think of a really lean, sleek, sexy hard body that's not big and bulky- that's what we are going for.

Resistance training means adding resistance to a motion and that could be in the form of water, tubing, weights, another person, or even wind! I go rollerblading at the beach, and windy days are hard work because the wind is giving resistance. I'm not just gliding anymore, now I'm really using muscle to push through that wind. This is not the ideal resistance training workout, but I just want to demonstrate that resistance training does not necessarily mean weights.

In the circumference of your body parts from outside to inside, you have skin, fat, and then muscle. If you just lose the fat in between the skin and muscle, you're still going to have a flabby muscle underneath saggy skin, and you won't be increasing your metabolism, in fact you will be decreasing it. Our goal here is to increase your body's need for calories and have a firm, tight arm, leg, or waist. Body type, age, and hormone levels will also play a role in how much muscle you have, how quickly the body adapts, and how that looks when it builds.

Building muscle means you get to eat more. Don't know about you, but I am not one who wants to keep eating less and less every year that I get older because I lose hormones, muscle, and metabolism. In fact, I want it to be quite the opposite. I love food and I want to keep enjoying what I love.

MYTH #2: DO CARDIO TO BURN FAT

Can you lose fat doing cardio? Absolutely, but is it guaranteed and is it the best way? Not necessarily. One of my very first clients, when I moved to California from New York, really wanted to lose weight. She was about 5-foot tall and started doing the treadmill and monitoring her calories. She was eating about a thousand calories a day, and she was doing an hour on the treadmill, five days a week. She called me because she was frustrated that she had only lost 5 pounds in 3 months.

Because she was over 50 and her hormones were changing, she was doing the wrong exercise. During menopause and andropause (the male version of menopause), you lose hormones that support keeping the muscle that you have. Even if you aren't 50 and you're not doing resistance training, you're still going to lose muscle every year after ages of 35.

She wasn't increasing her metabolism because she wasn't adding active tissue. Most women, especially over 50 think that, "In order to burn fat, I have to do cardio." The best scenario for you to burn fat is to increase your body's ability to burn fat by adding active tissue (build muscle), and that's by using resistance training, not by doing cardio.

Resistance training is like your long-term investment strategy, where cardio is your short term. You're not going to see the results right away with resistance training. Building muscle takes some time. However, once the body adapts, you can get results quickly.

Almost fifteen years ago, my company had a young woman client in her late twenties who worked out three days a week with us. She was monitoring her food (this was back before I was Paleo), and she only lost a pound or two in the first month. By the 8- or 9-week mark, seven pounds came right off. Nothing had changed about her food or program; her body adapted to the increased muscle and changed her metabolism. She had built muscle and lost some body fat. However, it's not like calories in and calories out- even back then we were not encouraging people to count every calorie. Your body is not a math equation- it's a chemistry lab.

MYTH #3: CARDIO INCREASES METABOLISM

This one is fun because in one way it is true- while you are exercising, cardio will increase your *working metabolism*. You will burn more calories by adding exercise. On the other hand, cardio does not increase *resting metabolism* and that is what we want for easy weight loss and weight management as we age. Even when you lose weight, you decrease your metabolism because it takes less energy to move a lighter person. Compare the energy needed to move a 200-pound person versus a 100-pound person. As you become lighter, you need less energy to move your lighter body- your gas tank shrinks. Ideally, we want to lose fat, build muscle, and maintain a higher metabolism. The only way to increase your metabolism and lose weight is to do resistance training and build muscle.

MYTH #4: JUST EXERCISE MORE

Not all exercise is equal. Think back to either a doctor telling you or someone else's advice, "just exercise more". Stop and think for a second-do you know specifically what to do with that information?

If I just said, "I would like you to go shopping," what does that mean? That brings up several questions. What kind of shopping? Let's say you're shopping for a dress. The next question would be what's the dress for? Is it a formal event? It is a casual event? Is it a cocktail dress? Is it an evening gown? The next question after that would be what time of year is it? Do I need long sleeves or short sleeves? Is it going to be hot or cool? All of these questions are natural to come up after someone gives you a very general recommendation.

Exercise is used often as a prescription for people in a way that's very general. I need a little bit more information than *just exercise*. Because we don't really talk about the different effects of exercise on your body, people are just looking for weight loss and are considering all exercise equal. That's one of the biggest myths because whether it's yoga, Pilates, a walk down the street, CrossFit, or training for a triathlon, they're all going to have different effects on your body.

MYTH #5: FIND EXERCISE YOU ENJOY

While preference is important for when you start, because not all exercise is equal, you might get frustrated that the exercise you enjoy is not getting you the results you want. I have been amazed at some of my favorite famous medical and health women who have the smallest chapters in their books about exercise! There is as much science to exercise as there is about nutrition, hormones, and general health.

The typical person might say, "Well, I don't like this kind of exercise, I only like that". Let's say it is walking or yoga. Anytime you start moving more than you did before there is a chance of seeing some results in the first 30-60 days. However, after your body adapts, you will plateau. Then you will wonder why you're not losing any weight because you didn't understand what to expect from yoga and walking. I have met people who have exercised five days a week who get no results before I see them, and then we make it three days a week and they get results. It's not necessarily the number of days that you're doing exercise; it boils down to the efficiency and effectiveness of what you are choosing to do and then how you do it.

MYTH #6: EXERCISE TO EAT WHATEVER YOU WANT

"If I do all this cardio, workout or hike and burn all these calories, now I can eat what I want because I've burned it away." If you are calorie counting, this might make sense to you. Just like, not all exercise is equal, neither are calories. We covered this in Chapter 7; so hopefully, by now you understand this on a new level. Foods like gluten, dairy, and sugar cause inflammation and water retention so even if you are eating fewer calories from these foods, having them in your diet can represent pounds of water retention and inflammation.

MYTH #7: GOING TO THE GYM ISN'T NATURAL

We have over 300 muscles and over 200 bones, and that's because we were designed to move, not sit. In our day and age, we do a lot of sitting and not a lot of motion. We don't hunt our food; we don't manually start fires to cook our food and warm ourselves; we're not building our own houses, so we're not actively doing what we're built to do and we forget that.

If we didn't have electricity, we'd all be very thin- same for technology. I'm not saying shut off all your lights when the sun goes down and live a caveman lifestyle in today's world, but remembering that our bodies are designed to be moving and active can encourage you to look for more ways to use your body.

I'm that crazy friend that helps people move, and I do it because it's a great exercise opportunity, whereas most of my friends think I'm nuts when I ask them to help me. I actually like taking a heavy set of boxes up two flights of stairs because that will be my work out for the day. Walking up the stairs with weights (boxes) in my hands is the equivalent of doing lunges.

Manual labor, such as cleaning the house, is also exercise. I had heard a story told by the late Dr. Wayne Dyer that cited a study done on hotel housekeepers. They divided the staff into two groups: one group was made aware that their job was exercise and the others were not instructed any particular way. They found that after a period of time, the group that was made aware that their job was exercise lost weight while the other group did not.

I don't normally clean a lot, but when I clean for events, I wear a heart rate monitor because I want to know how many calories I burned, how efficient my time was, and how hard was I working. Not because I'm going to eat them back but because I'm showing myself that my daily chores or working in the yard is exercise.

The limiting belief many people have is to think of exercise as "I'm trapped in the gym like a rat. I have to do the treadmill so

I don't gain weight, because I'm going to eat these things later." As long as you stay in that mentality with exercise and the gym, your relationship to exercise isn't a healthy one.

If we were to reverse that a little bit, I would recommend taking a different approach to exercise, giving your body an opportunity to be in use. Everyday ask yourself, "What did I do with all my muscles and bones, did I use any of them? How many of them did I use? Where could I use them that would benefit me and my body?"

For instance, I live close enough to the bank that if I'm working from home, I will walk to the bank to deposit a check versus drive to the bank, because I'm getting exercise while completing a task. I'm combining a task that I want to complete with a task that I have to complete.

If you have no activities or manual labor to complete on a regular basis, the gym provides you tools to work your 300+ muscles and 200+ bones. Moreover, most manual labor will not be able to give attention to all your muscles and you will need to balance your body with working on opposite muscles to provide balance, support, and avoid injury.

MYTH #8: THE GYM IS THE BEST WORKOUT

The best workouts start with the workout you will do. The next best workout to start is the one designed to get you results with resistance training and heart rate targeted cardio or interval training for your specific body and fitness level.

None of that has to happen in the gym. I teach people how to exercise in their home because people don't understand the tools that they have access to all the time. When you learn about your muscles and proper exercise, you realize you can do it almost anywhere.

The key isn't how much weight you are using or a specific machine, it's whether or not it's the appropriate amount of force and intensity to get you results. We use body weight as resistance as well as hand weights, ankle weights, and elastic tubing. A bag of resistance tubing with all of its parts weighs a pound or two and you can take it with you, secure the door anchor, and work the entire body.

The myth about getting a better workout at the gym stops people from working out. When you understand how to utilize small objects that travel easily, rather than telling yourself, "I don't have time to go to the gym," you can say, "Oh, I have 10 minutes in between this thing and that thing where I can do some exercise." Rather than making the excuse of why you can't do it, create ways to get it in.

MYTH #9: EXERCISE TAKES TOO MUCH TIME

First, there is the question of your goals, then, focus on how to create an effective program that is also time efficient. When we generalize how long exercise will take without specifying it to our personal needs and schedule, it's easy to use this as excuse. One of my clients has lost 100 pounds working out twice a week for the last few years. Because of her job, she does not have many days to commit to exercise so we created her program only exercising 2 days a week. We will go over the formula for creating your program in the next chapter.

MYTH #10: SOMETHING IS BETTER THAN NOTHING

Generally this is true, moving is better than not moving. The myth comes into play when you think any and all moving is exercise that will make changes in your body. There is one word I want you to learn that can change your workouts- adaptation. This is when your body changes in accordance with the demands you are placing on it. Let's say you start a walking program, with no heart rate monitor tracking, three days a week for thirty minutes after doing no exercise for many years. Within a few weeks, your body will build a little muscle, gain a little flexibility, and increase endurance. There might not be any weight loss but there has been adaptation. Because the body is now stronger and lighter, it does not need to change anymore for this kind of exercise. Most people plateau, get frustrated, and quit exercising because of the lack of results after the initial adaptation. Same thing goes for a very disciplined person who has been doing the same exact program for years; while committing to doing the exercise keeps you at your health level, it stopped making changes in your body a long time ago. Every time the body adapts to the exercise you are doing, there is a need to change the intensity or type of exercise in order to keep stimulating change in your body.

CHAPTER 8

BUILD THE PROGRAM

"By failing to prepare, you are preparing to fail ."

Benjamin Franklin

W E'RE GOING TO USE the FITT principle; the top graph on the following page will be for cardiovascular activities and the bottom for resistance training. Cardio would be walking, running, hiking, biking, swimming, dancing, aerobics class, boxing, kickboxing, and activities at a low intensity that you could sustain for longer periods of time. Resistance training can mean lifting weights, but also using body weight or workout tubing. However, certain kinds of yoga, certain moves in Pilates, and some boxing and kickboxing can be considered resistance training. Resistance training is adding force in the opposite direction to your motion that is intense enough for your muscles that you could not continue to do the same motion for more than 90 seconds without rest.

This chapter also has an audio version and the FITT principle worksheet can be downloaded and printed every time you hit a plateau and need to adjust your workout program. Visit *invisiblefitness.com* to download the free audio and worksheet. Stat by filling out the topic row of both of the graphs.

1. "F" stands for Frequency- Write down how many days a week you engage in cardio or how many times a week. If you walk a couple of blocks to get to work, and that's all you do, we can consider it cardio. If you exercise and then walk a few places, I wouldn't consider that cardio. Now go into the "F" under the resistance training and write down how many days of the week you do resistance training of any kind, even doing some abs, if you do crunches, can be considered resistance training.

2. "I" stands for Intensity-there are two ways to gauge intensity. The first way is called the rate of perceived exertion (RPE). On a scale of 1 to 10, rate how hard the exercise is for you, 1 being sitting at your desk, or lying on the bed, and 5 being something that's 50% of effort. The more effective way to test your intensity level would be with a heart rate monitor. Having a heart rate monitor is important for judging correctly the efficiency and the effectiveness of a cardio workout. Rate yourself for cardiovascular work first then jump down to the resistance training and do the same thing. For resistance training, an RPE of 10 would be lifting to controlled failure. Failure means you are giving 100% effort and not moving anymore. If you feel your resistance training 2 days later in the muscles that you worked, it may be a 7-9. If you feel no soreness or fatigue at all a day or two later, it's probably more of a 5-6.

F= Frequency, I= Intensity, T= Time, T= Type

Cardio

F	I	T	T

Resistance Training

F	I	T	T

3. The first "T" is Time. How much time do you spend working out? Is it a range between 10 minutes and 20 minutes? Is it a range between 30 and an hour? Even if you do different times for different machines or activities, list it all, same thing with resistance. If you do crunches,

push-ups, or anything like that, and you're counting that as resistance, which it is, and it might only be five minutes. Don't count the length of time you are at the gym, only the time you are actually exercising.

4. The second "T" is Type. What kind of exercise do you do? For cardio, you can refer to the list at the beginning of this chapter and list all the different machines or types of cardio you are doing. For resistance training, you can list all the exercises or machines you are doing. Having a professional help you create this will get you better results but at least you can start with where you are and build from there.

After you have all the top row of boxes on both charts filled out, ask, "Is it working?" If you are getting results, then keep doing what you're doing until you hit a plateau. When you start to feel like you're not getting results anymore, then you have to look at which one or two of these factors to change. The second row of boxes is for you to write in where you will make adjustments. This is the formula that you can keep using to keep getting results. Create a new chart every time you start something new or get to a new level of fitness, lifestyle or age.

THE IMPORTANCE OF HEART RATE

Knowing and tracking your heart rate gives you a lot of information that you would otherwise miss. First, a decrease in your heart rate on an activity that you have been doing regularly shows your first sign of cardiovascular improvement. It's the first sign that your heart is stronger; you improved your strength and endurance. Most importantly, it often happens before you see major weight loss. If you aren't tracking it, you could be frustrated too early and think that your exercise is not working.

Secondly, it's an important safety reading so you can know what's going on inside your body when there are no other signs. Many years ago, I was trying to teach a friend of mine how to rollerblade. The first mistake I made was expecting to get a good workout at the same time. I was fearful that she wasn't going to be fast enough to keep my heart rate in my target heart rate zone. Five minutes into the rollerblade, my heart rate spiked to 183. The top of my zone at the time was 190, so 183 was high for the amount of effort I was putting forth. I wasn't going that fast and so I was a bit concerned. When we got back from rollerblading, I put a thermometer in my mouth and found out that I had a fever. The heart monitor isn't just to burn calories and track where you are going. When your mind says you want to finish or accomplish a task, it's allowing you to see what your body is telling you, in case you're not paying attention. I had a fever and I was really happy I didn't push myself any harder because it could have resulted in more serious side effects.

Next, knowing your target heart rate helps you to be more efficient with your time and to choose exercises that are the appropriate intensity. As your body adapts, you will need to increase either your time or intensity. Too often people start to plateau and do not have the understanding of how to make the next best modification to keep getting results.

Not only can monitoring your heart rate get you results and keep you safe, it is also a great motivational tool. When I first started working with "Nancy" in Florida, one of my clients on the 90-Day Health and Body Makeover, she was doing many yoga classes. She wanted to lose a couple more pounds, so I had her wear the heart monitor during both her Bikrum and Hatha yoga classes each week. We discovered that in an hour and a half long class, she was in her zone for zero minutes of those ninety minutes. Yoga is not necessarily a good choice for cardio but she was shocked to see how inefficient yoga was for getting her to her goals and how much time she was spending a week in classes. Most people assume if they sweat, that must have meant a good workout, and that's not necessarily true. As your fitness level increases, so does the need for more intensity. The zone won't change, what you need to do to get into it will.

Using heart rate training can also cut your workout time in half. I had an attorney client who was on a medical weight loss program and was spending four hours a week on a recumbent bike. He had results because of his drastic diet changes and some medications but when he stopped the drugs and the diet, he gained it all back, even though he never stopped doing the bike. When he met with me, the first thing I looked at was his efficiency. Once we strapped the heart rate monitor on him and figured out his target heart rate zone, we discovered that he was only efficient for 15 minutes out of an hour, which equals one hour out of four hours. That whole week he wasted three hours. This is a situation where my recommendation was to cut the time in half and increase the intensity by 50% or more. Using a heart rate monitor allowed him to get more results in half the time.

WHY PASSIVE STRETCHING IS DANGEROUS

This could have gone under the myth section but I thought the topic of stretching deserved more explanation. I have several videos where I explain this and use the visual of my own body as an example so if you find it difficult to visualize here, please visit jjflizanes.tv to find the Smart Exercise Playlist and the video titled, " Why Passive Stretching is Dangerous". There are two main types of stretching, active and passive. Passive stretching can injure you and does not increase active range of motion.

First, let me ask you, where did you learn how to stretch? Many people learned in high school, junior high or on a sports team from a "coach" who was your math teacher during the day. Maybe they studied biology, but not specifically biomechanics, anatomy, physiology, and definitely not on this particular subject of stretching.

I want you to visualize a muscle like Velcro and as the muscle contracts and pulls together, what happens is something called cross bridging. Imagining Velcro, the cross bridging is what's pulling the muscle together and shortens it. This is a very strong position. You have all of this cross bridging, or let's say Velcro that's connected. As it starts to stretch and lengthen, it loses its strength because it loses the cross bridging. There will be certain point where there's no longer any cross bridging, which means there's no neurological control from your brain to your muscle.

Once there's no longer any cross bridging in the muscle, it is in a complete stretch and it leaves the muscle susceptible to be torn. In this lengthened position, this muscle no longer is moving and no longer active. It's sleeping, so to speak. In order for a muscle to get like this, some other muscle has to be pulling it there.

All your muscles are synergistic. So let's take the biceps for instance. When the biceps contracts, the triceps stretch. I can't shorten my biceps and triceps at the same time. When my triceps contract, my biceps stretch. Now you understand that every muscle in the body has a synergistic relationship with the opposite muscle. When one is contracting, the other one is stretching.

Why are you stretching in the first place? What is the point of stretching? Most people think that stretching allows them to move further, increase range of motion. Let's say, for instance, I want to be able to pull my shoulders back further behind me, and I want to be able to stretch my chest further. Well, in order to do that, some muscle has to be contracting. The "stretched muscle" that has no cross bridging doesn't do anything.

Relaxed muscles do not move bone, contracted muscles move bone. If you want to increase your range of motion, concentrate on the muscles that are pulling you into that position, not on the ones that are relaxed, doing nothing. This would be considered active stretching. If you have a well-rounded resistance-training program, all the muscles that are worked are also stretched within a balanced program

An example of a common injury with passive stretching happens in the hamstrings. Imagine lying down on your back and using only your quadriceps muscles (front thigh) to pull your leg towards you. As an active stretch, your thigh muscles will have a certain range of how far they can lift/pull your leg towards your head. This is your active range of motion, the limit you currently have of muscle strength and ability to relax your hamstring muscles (back of thigh).

What trainers and most people teach you to do at this point, is to use your hands and arms to pull your leg closer to your body- this is a passive stretch. The increase of range of motion is now dictated by how hard you pull your leg towards you, not on the current ability of your leg muscles, which are your target. Many trainers, and I am guilty of this in earlier years too, use their body weight to push against your leg in the air and move it closer to you. If the pressure applied is more than your muscle can handle, it will tear. This is the same for every muscle in your body that needs an external force to move it further than it can by itself. Another very beneficial video to watch is called, "All Muscles Pull, Not Push", which you can find in the Smart Exercise Playlist or even on the video podcast on iTunes. Passive stretching does not increase your active range of motion. It may feel good, which is why people do it but just be aware that it does not have as much benefit as active stretching and can damage your body and decrease your strength capabilities over time.

CHAPTER 9

SECRET 3: BALANCE AND REPLENISH HORMONES

"The inferior physician treats advanced disease.
The mediocre physician treats early disease. The
superior physician prevents disease ."

Chinese proverb

SINCE 2007, I HAVE BEEN working with The Nourishing Wellness Medical Center, an Age Management Practice that focuses on helping patients to live a longer, healthier, and more vital life. Owned by Dr. Allen Peters and Jeanne Peters RD, for many years we were a triangle approach to a complete health regime. Doc Allen would focus on hormones, Jeanne looked at nutrition, and I addressed the exercise piece. For over ten years, I have been in the front of the class learning about hormones from Doc Allen and Jeanne, as well as other physicians I have featured on the Fit 2 Love Podcast Show who have also researched and studied hormones extensively, like Dr. Elizabeth Plourde.

Hormone health is what regulates so many of our processes. There's a huge connection between our hormone health, keeping it at optimal levels, and our overall systemic health. If one thing is out of balance, over time, many of the different hormone patterns can get out of balance. We have endocrine hormones that regulate our blood sugars and growth patterns. Human growth hormone is essential for helping to maximize muscle mass which effects your metabolism and ability to burn fat. Hormones like insulin are responsible for helping to absorb the sugar that you generate from your foods. Then you have sex hormones, which are not only just available to help with your libido, but also to keep your bones and brain strong. There are receptor sites for testosterone, progesterone, and estrogen in our brains.

We're biochemically altered when these hormones are low or removed from us, and that alters our neurotransmitters, and how we feel. That alters our serotonin. Estradiol is essential for us to be able to produce serotonin, and serotonin is what makes us feel good. When our hormones are depleted or out of balance, it can also cause weight loss resistance. Even with proper nutrition and exercise, the body will not respond optimally because the chemistry is off. Most Western physicians are starting to add comprehensive hormone labs into their practices but mainstream medicine is slow to acknowledge the effects of these hormones on aging as well as weight gain, depression, sleeplessness, anxiety, joint, and bone injuries.

Dr. Elizabeth Plourde, after a hysterectomy, got osteoarthritis in her hands so bad they looked horrible and misshapen. She had enlarged joints, and her fingers were all angled over. Her joints were so painful she couldn't even open jars. She finally got hormones that her body could absorb and within four months, the pain had gone away, and within two years, her joints were all back to natural size. All of our joints and ligaments need hormones.

Imagine a three-sided triangle and each of the parts of the triangle equal in length and distance. On the first side are the sex hormones, second side are thyroid hormones and the third side are the stress hormones. Let's assume that you are the average American making career decisions, not getting enough sleep, the diet is not great, but you work out hard. In order to be able to manage and maintain your stress hormones, like DHEA, it might steal from your progesterone or testosterone and convert those sex hormones into stress hormones. The body, like Legos, can break apart, make something new with it, and learn to adapt. One of the ways that might impact a woman who has high stress is that her progesterone levels will begin to fall. In this scenario, she's going to have some PMS issues right around the time of her ovulation and period. When the stress hormones are out of balance, the body starts stealing from the sex hormones, and then ultimately can throw off the thyroid.

This is where stress can start us on a track to metabolic syndrome, aka weight loss resistance, which leads to insulin resistance, hypertension, high cholesterol, and diabetes. Now you have a very serious medical problem that if you don't prevent, it's very difficult to treat.

"Physicians are trained to treat disease with medications and surgery, they are not trained as preventive practitioners"

Dr. Allen Peters.

AVOID HYSTERECTOMY

Medical doctors are told that, "These organs are only for childbearing, they're useless. You don't need them anymore."

They have counseled women for the last century saying that this is the case once you've past childbearing years; all they are is just places for cancers to grow. Ten percent of the hysterectomies or the uterus removal is for cancer and only five percent of the ovary removal is for cancer. The others, there's answers for any of the other conditions.

We want to encourage the preservation of these organs as much as possible because they do so much for the body. Dr. Elizabeth Plourde's book, **Hysterectomy, Ovary Removal, and Hormone Replacement: What All Women Needto Know** isessential because you really need to understand what these organs are doing for us. They're not just for childbearing; they are integral in the structure of the pelvic area. Women have a lot of bladder problems (the bladder is falling down) and vaginal prolapse, when these organs are removed. The other thing that they're never warned of is that, the ligaments that hold the uterus are the strongest in the body. You cut those and you really allow the whole back to start collapsing because you've lost a lot of support. I was able to interview Dr. Plourde several times on my podcast show and she strongly recommends many other methods rather than removal. She agreed that cancer is a reason for removing, but the last time she looked at the 625,000 hysterectomies in the United States, and half a million of those, including the ovary removal, were because women are told, "Oh, gee, you don't need them," when in reality, after menopause, those ovaries still keep producing valuable testosterone. Testicles don't shut down creating testosterone, and neither do the ovaries. It's really a myth that the ovaries shut down at menopause. Testosterone is very valuable. It goes into the brain, is converted into estradiol, which is our pre-menopausal estrogen, and it is very protective against Alzheimer's disease. One of the many reasons that more women have Alzheimer's disease is because we have so much less estradiol. We have none after menopause, and then we only have it when the testosterone goes into the brain cells and is converted into estradiol. Whereas men have a lot more testosterone than we do, so they're constantly protecting their brain against Alzheimer's disease.

Dr. Plourde had serious health concerns after she was convinced to have a hysterectomy, which sent her researching background on a mission to solve her problem and understand what was going on. One of her first symptoms was bladder incontinence, because the urethra of the bladder actually needs to have estrogen. Women deserve to know that estrogen and testosterone are the answer, because we need the strength in the muscles. We absolutely have to have testosterone in order to have muscle strength for our entire body and spine. We start deteriorating completely without these hormones in our body, and we're being told, "Oh, they're dangerous. Don't take them. They cause breast cancer." Well, the end result is osteoporosis, un-mendable broken hip, and being in a nursing home. When we have these hormones in our body, we are much healthier because they're designed to be there. Many women are suffering needlessly with Alzheimer's disease, osteoporosis, muscle weakness, or arthritis.

When working with Nourishing Wellness patients or Invisible Fitness clients who are tested for all of these, I always encourage my clients to understand their bloodwork and to ask for tests that may give them more information. I want you to have that same understanding so you can be proactive and preventative to your health and aging. You can download the list of hormones that I cover here at *invisiblefitness.com* to start the conversation with your doctor or to find a preventative, age management physician who will work with you. Hormones are Secret 3 in this process because the majority of people struggling with releasing weight have hormonal imbalances causing an obstacle to weight loss goals. The first set of hormones to address make up your adrenals and are considered stress hormones. We have an epidemic of adrenal fatigue and this step is the easiest and fastest to self-correct.

ADRENAL FATIGUE

This commonly undiagnosed epidemic, that I have experienced first-hand several times, can also be known casually as burn out. Your adrenal glands produce a variety of hormones that are essential to life. The medical term adrenal insufficiency (or Addison's disease) refers to inadequate production of one or more of these hormones as a result of an underlying disease. Many people don't hear about it because, unfortunately, traditional medicine still doesn't necessarily acknowledge it. However, functional medicine and functional nutrition does because we are looking at the function of the body. The adrenal glands are two little almond-shaped glands that sit on top of the kidneys and regulate your stress hormones, which include cortisol and DHEA. Adrenal insufficiency can be diagnosed by blood tests that show inadequate levels of adrenal hormones. Functional medicine sees this as a mild form of adrenal insufficiency caused by chronic stress because the adrenal glands are unable to keep pace with the demands of perpetual fight-or-flight experiences. Work with a physician to test cortisol and DHEA.

CORTISOL

Cortisol is a stress hormone that circulates during the day. Its primary function is to help support the energy demands of the body and liberate sugar and fuel into your bloodstream. If you're somebody who's pushing your body beyond its limits and putting out plenty of cortisol during the day, you may not be replenishing at night during sleep when sleep is most essential for our hormone health. Over time, you may find that your adrenal glands aren't responding as well, and not producing enough of these critical hormones to be able to sustain balanced energy.

WHAT CORTISOL DOES

» Mobilizes and increases amino acids, the building blocks of protein, in the blood and liver

» Stimulates the liver to convert amino acids to glucose, the primary fuel for energy production

» Stimulates increased glycogen in the liver (Glycogen is the stored form of glucose)

» Mobilizes and increases fatty acids in the blood (from fat cells) to be used as fuel for energy production

» Counteracts inflammation and allergies

» Prevents the loss of sodium in urine and thus helps maintain blood volume and blood pressure

» Maintains resistance to stress (e.g. infections, physical trauma, temperature extremes, emotional trauma, etc.)

» Maintains mood and emotional stability

» Excess Cortisol

» Diminishes cellular utilization of glucose

» Increases blood sugar levels

» Decreases protein synthesis

» Increases protein breakdown that can lead to muscle wasting

» Causes demineralization of bone that can lead to osteoporosis

» Interferes with skin regeneration and healing

» Causes shrinking of lymphatic tissue

» Diminishes lymphocyte numbers and functions

» Lessens SIgA (secretory antibody productions), this immune system suppression may lead to increased susceptibility to allergies, infections, and degenerative disease

DHEA (DEHYDROEPIANDROSTERONE)

DHEA, the second stress hormones, is the precursor for testosterone, which is the precursor for estrogen. DHEA is a mother hormone that helps your body make your sex and thyroid hormones. DHEA is an anti-stress hormone, so it's very important on its own and it's important as a precursor.

FUNCTIONS OF DHEA

» Functions as an androgen (a male hormone) with anabolic activity, "Anabolic" refers to the building or synthesis of tissues

» Is a precursor that is converted to testosterone (a male hormone), and is a precursor to estrogen (a female anabolic hormone)

» Reverses immune suppression caused by excess cortisol levels, thereby improving resistance against viruses, bacteria and *Candida albicans*, parasites, allergies, and cancer

» Stimulates bone deposition and remodeling to prevent osteoporosis

» Improves cardiovascular status by lowering total cholesterol and LDL levels, thereby lessening incidences of heart attack

» Increases muscle mass and decreases percentage of body fat

» Involved in the thyroid gland's conversion of the less active T4 to the more active T3

» Reverses many of the unfavorable effects of excess cortisol, creating subsequent improvement in energy/vitality, sleep, premenstrual symptoms, and mental clarity

» Accelerates recovery from any kind of acute stress (e.g. insufficient sleep, excessive exercise, mental strain, etc.)

COMMON CAUSES OF ADRENAL STRESS

» Anger

» Fear

» Worry/anxiety

» Depression

» Guilt

» Overwork/physical or mental strain

» Excessive exercise

» Sleep deprivation

» Going to sleep late

» Surgery

» Trauma/injury

» Chronic inflammation

» Chronic infection

» Chronic pain

» Temperature extremes

» Toxic exposure

» Nutritional deficiencies

» Chronic illness

» Chronic-severe allergies

ASSOCIATED SYMPTOMS AND CONSEQUENCES OF IMPAIRED ADRENALS

» Low body temperature

» Nervousness

» Mental depression

» Hypoglycemia

» Tendency towards inflammation

» Poor memory

» Osteoporosis

» Lightheadedness

» Poor resistance to infections

» Food allergies & Environmental allergies

» Dry and thin skin

» Weakness

» Unexplained hair loss

» Difficulty building muscle

» Irritability

» Difficulty gaining weight

» Apprehension

» Inability to concentrate

» Excessive hunger

» Moments of confusion

» Indigestion

» Digestive Stress

» Auto-immune hepatitis

» Auto-immune diseases

» Palpitations

» Dizziness

» Low blood pressure

» Insomnia

» PMS

» Craving for sweets

» Headaches

STRESS REDUCTION TO IMPROVE ADRENAL HORMONES NATURALLY

» Regular physical activity

» Meditation

» Mindfulness and breath work

» Yoga

» Social connectedness

» Laughter

» Spend time in nature

» Music

» Have more fun

» EFT: Emotional Freedom Techniques

CHAPTER 10

THE ORCHESTRA OF SEX HORMONES

"It's not enough to add years to one's life... one
must add life to those years ."

John F. Kennedy

THE LIFE FORCE that fuels metabolism, the ability to build active tissue, and increase energy expenditure are your hormones. Hormone replacement and balancing is restoration, and restoration stops deterioration. Paying attention to your sex hormones is important at every age for optimal health. In the last forty years, testosterone has decreased in men by 100 milligrams on average and it's starting as early for men in their late thirties. In recent years, researchers have noticed general links between low testosterone and other medical conditions. A comprehensive investigation of people's metabolism is necessary in order to achieve the results that you desire.

TESTOSTERONE

Testosterone is a hormone that acts as the primary sex hormone in men. It is produced by the male testicles and the female ovaries. Testosterone levels, in men, increase during and after puberty, dropping after about age 40.

FUNCTIONS OF TESTOSTERONE

» Anabolic- build tissues

» Increases libido

» Increases muscle strength

» Increase bone density

» Decrease inflammation

» Improves energy

» Lower LDL

» Raise HDL

» Enhance blood glucose levels

» Improves Brain function

» Decrease Body Fat

» Increases Heart Strength

LOW TESTOSTERONE

» Fatigue

» Memory loss

» Abdominal fat

» Weight gain

HIGH TESTOSTERONE

» Chin hairs

» Oily skin

» Acne

» Scalp hair loss

» Unwanted body hair

» Aggressive behavior

» Sugar or Salt Cravings

ESTROGEN

Estrogen is the primary female sex hormone and is responsible for the development and regulation of the female reproductive system, and secondary sex characteristics. Estrogen is an entire class of related hormones that includes estriol, estradiol, and estrone and about thirty other estrogens. Beginning at puberty, a woman's ovaries start releasing estrogen in coordination with each monthly menstrual cycle. At mid-cycle, levels suddenly spike, triggering the release of an egg (ovulation). During the rest of the month, estrogen levels climb and fall gradually, so normal estrogen levels vary widely. Estrogen must be balanced with progesterone and each person will have different needs.

ESTROGEN AFFECTS:

» Brain

» Liver

» Bones

» Skin

» Uterus

» Urinary tract

» Breasts

» Eye Membranes

» Blood vessels

» Emotional well being

» Increasing serotonin, and the number of serotonin receptors in the brain

» Modifying the production and the effects of endorphins, the "feel-good" chemicals in the brain

» Protecting nerves from damage, and possibly stimulating nerve growth

LOW ESTROGEN

» Unexplained Weight Gain

» Bloating

» Itching

» Sweating

» Hot Flashes

» Bladder Infections

» Depression

» Fatigue

» Heart Palpitations

» Weight gain

PROGESTERONE

Progesterone is a hormone that occurs naturally in the body released by the ovaries and adrenal glands. Changing progesterone levels can contribute to abnormal menstrual periods and menopausal symptoms. Progesterone is also necessary for implantation of the fertilized egg in the uterus and for maintaining pregnancy.

FUNCTIONS OF PROGESTERONE:

» Repairs and maintains a healthy brain

» Calming effect

» Builds bone

» Natural diuretic

» Burns Fat

» Helps Prevent Cancer

» Balances Estrogen

» Low Progesterone:

» Sleep Disturbances

» Irritability

» Anxiety

» Weight Gain

» Breast Swelling

» Breast Tenderness

» Itching

» Bloating

» Sweating

» Loss of Memory

» Loss of Libido

THYROID HORMONES

The thyroid-stimulating hormone comes from your brain to activate two hormones called, T3 and T4. It regulates your overall ability to transform energy into heat energy, many things can affect thyroid. Most people get the TSH tested but not T3 and T4. Some doctors are now recognizing that we probably ought to change our levels of thyroid. Right now, a typical range of thyroid would be .5 to 4.5--which is a big range. There are many people that are walking around that may be under a physician's guide who may be saying there is no thyroid issue, but actually, they would do better if they could optimize those levels into a lower range. It's a butterfly shaped gland below the Adam's Apple. Thyroid is a major contributor to metabolism and can induce weight gain when it is slightly off, with no change in diet. The major three thyroid tests to get are TSH, T3 and T4. The thyroid hormones are composed of three or four iodine molecules, so you will want to make sure you have a good source of iodine as well.

FUNCTIONS OF THYROID:

» Metabolism

» Body Temperate

» Cell Energy Production

» Proper function and maturation of all other hormones

LOW THYROID

» Susceptibility to infection

» Swelling, usually in face

» Thickening skin

» Chronic Pain

» Fatigue

» Dry Skin

» High Blood Pressure

» Irregular Heart Beat

» Sleep Apnea

» Sensitivity to hot and cold

» Unexplained Weight Gain

» Missing outer third of eyebrows

» Constipation

» Repeated infections

» Brittle Nails

» Hair Loss

» Intolerance to heat

» Muscle Weakness

» Low Blood Pressure

» Osteoporosis

» Joint/Muscle Pain

» Cystic breasts

» Chronic sinusitis

» Asthma

» And more!

TSH- THYROID STIMULATING HORMONE

TSH is a hormone produced by your master gland, the pituitary. The higher it is the more stimulation it provides. It serves a negative feedback loop to the thyroid. Therefore, when TSH levels are low, it means the thyroid is generally producing enough thyroid hormone. When TSH levels are high, this usually means the body requires more thyroid hormone.

T3- TRIIODOTHYRONINE

Triiodothyronine or T3 is critically important because it tells the nucleus of your cells to send messages to your DNA to rev up your metabolism by burning fat. This is how T3 lowers cholesterol levels, regrows hair, and helps keep you lean. T3 levels can be disrupted by nutritional imbalances, toxins, allergens, infections, and stress, and this leads to a series of complications, including thyroid cancer, hypothyroidism, and hyperthyroidism, which today are three of the most prevalent thyroid-related diseases.

T4- THYROXINE

Many of your cells and tissues depend on thyroxine, T4, to work properly. An overactive thyroid secretes too much T4, causing some of your body functions to accelerate. Physicians may use the term, "thyrotoxicosis" instead of "hyperthyroidism." This condition is more common in women – about eight in 100 women and one in 100 men develop hyperthyroidism at some point in their lives.

BELLY FAT AND HORMONES

Adipose tissue, visceral fat, is actually an active organ. Dr. Mark Houston, out of the University of Vanderbilt, addresses that the adipose tissue is not only an active organ but also it's a damaging active organ. It's s putting out inflammatory markers, multiple cytokines, which are extremely inflammatory towards every organ in your body. Adipose tissue also secretes low-density lipo protein and excess estrogen, which is not necessarily bad but can be, in excess, in both men and women.

As you create more inflammation, you have more weight loss resistance; the more weight loss resistance, the greater deposits of adipose tissue. It becomes this vicious cycle increasing your obesity, inflammation, weight loss resistance and setting you up for metabolic syndrome. Inflammation is a major issue and most of it comes from your own adipose tissue.

BIOIDENTICAL HORMONES

There are two types of hormone replacement therapy on the market - HRT and BHRT. BHRT, Bio-Identical Hormone Replacement Therapy, has been around for 70 years with testosterone being the first to be produced successfully. Pharmaceutical companies then started making synthetic hormones (HRT) in order to patent them because bioidentical hormones can't be patented. Unfortunately, when they made them patentable, they introduced foreign substances into the production and therefore into the bodies of humans. The results, although initially appeared to be somewhat favorable, in the end could be extremely dangerous.

Common wisdom then decided to judge all hormones the same and consider them all dangerous. On the political side, pharmaceutical companies, who are donating billions of dollars to medical schools, do not want the medical schools teaching about bioidentical hormones. This is because a healthy 75-year-old, like Dr. Allen Peters, who takes bioidentical hormones, is not on the seven medications that the average 75-year-old is taking for high blood pressure, cholesterol, blood thinners, depression, and more. Functional and alternative medicine is up against a $500 billion dollar industry.

Bioidentical hormones are made from plants, and convert to being identical to what humans naturally produce. Mainstream medicine is catching on and they're using them more and more, especially in Europe. Unfortunately, most of the studies that have been done that create fear around hormone replacement therapy have been done with the premerine provera, the horse urine estrogens, and progesterone. Because they come from horse urine, they are not an identical match to what the human body produces. Studies show a mild increase in breast cancer with the synthetic hormones.

Yet even these synthetic hormones actually reduce incidences of colon cancer, which is the second most fatal cancer for men and third for women. More important than that is the reduction of osteoporosis and osteoporotic fractures. Do you know that the mortality of an osteoporotic fracture in a woman at three months is greater than the mortality of breast cancer in ten years? Hormone replacement therapy goes a long way towards preventing those fractures. We have one and a half million of those fractures every year, versus 50,000 people who die of breast cancer-not to diminish breast cancer but to put it in perspective. Bioidentical hormones are believed to be dramatically safer and provide a drastic reduction in chronic degenerative disease and aging. They improve the quality of life by optimizing and getting your hormones back to where they were when you were the most vigorous and vital. There can be a phenomenal increase in quality of life, as well as help with weight loss resistance by optimizing your hormones.

RECOMMENDED PREVENTIVE BLOODWORK LIST

» Testosterone

» Estrogen   } Sex Hormones

» Progesterone

» TSH

» T3   } Thyroid Hormones

» T4

» DHEA   } Adrenal/Stress Hormones

» Cortisol

» Vit D

» CRP

» A1C

» Iron

» Ferritin

» B12

CHAPTER 11

ADDITIONAL IMPORTANT MARKERS

"The part can never be well unless the whole is well ."

Plato

N OW THAT WE HAVE COVERED the major sex, stress, and thyroid hormones, there are a few more labs that would be good to test regularly. The full list can be downloaded at *www.invisiblefitness.com*

VITAMIN D

Vitamin D deficiency is incredibly common in the US, but many Americans mistakenly believe they aren't at risk because they consume vitamin-D-fortified foods (such as milk). There are very few foods that actually have therapeutic levels of vitamin D, naturally, and even fortified foods do not contain enough vitamin D to support your health needs. Despite its name, vitamin D is not a regular vitamin. It's actually a steroid hormone that you are designed to obtain primarily through sun exposure, not diet. Research into vitamin D over the past two decades has revealed a spectacular amount of solid evidence backing its importance for countless aspects of human health. A few years back, the recommended level was between, 4 to 60 nanograms per milliliter (ng/ml), but more recently the optimal vitamin D level has been raised to 50-70 ng/ml, and when treating cancer or heart disease, as high as 70-100 ng/ml. Because most people do not get enough sun exposure or optimal levels of vitamin D, there is a need to supplement it, to keep levels in the higher range.

SYMPTOMS OF VITAMIN D DEFICIENCY

» Darker skin

» Obesity

» Achy bones

» Feeling blue

» Head sweating

» Gut trouble

BENEFITS OF VITAMIN D

Vitamin D can aid in preventing cancer, heart disease, autoimmune diseases, infections, and mental health conditions. Vitamin D also fights infections, including colds and the flu, as it regulates the expression of genes that influence your immune system to attack and destroy bacteria and viruses.

Optimizing your vitamin D levels can help protect against:

» **Cardiovascular disease** - Vitamin D is very important for reducing hypertension, atherosclerotic heart disease, heart attack, and stroke. According to Dr. Michael Holick, Author of **The Vitamin D Solution,** one study showed that vitamin D deficiency increased the risk of heart attack by 50 percent.

» **Autoimmune diseases** - Vitamin D is a potent immune modulator, making it very important for the prevention of autoimmune diseases, like multiple sclerosis and inflammatory bowel disease.

» **Infections, including influenza** - It also helps you fight infections of all kinds. A study done in Japan, for example, showed that schoolchildren taking 1,200 units of vitamin D per day during winter reduced their risk of getting influenza by about 40 percent.

» **DNArepairandmetabolicprocesses** – One of Dr. Holick's studies showed that healthy volunteers taking 2,000 IUs of vitamin D per day for a few months upregulated 291 different genes that control up to 80 different metabolic processes, from improving DNA repair to having effect on boosting your immune system and many other biological processes.

C- REACTIVE PROTEIN

The body produces C-reactive protein, or CRP, when something is starting to become inflamed. High levels of CRP have been found to increase the risk of heart disease. CRP measures inflammation and is made in the liver and in cells lining blood vessels. Levels of the protein rise with factors that make heart disease more probable, such as obesity, smoking, diabetes, and high cholesterol. I think this is an important test that can help determine leaky gut and how diet affects digestion. Other reasons to have CRP tested are to identify and keep track of infections and diseases that cause inflammation, such as:

» Cancer of the lymph nodes (lymphoma)

» Diseases of the immune system, such as lupus

» Painful swelling of the blood vessels in the head and neck (giant cell arteritis)

» Painful swelling of the tissues that line the joints (rheumatoid arthritis)

» Swelling and bleeding of the intestines (inflammatory bowel disease)

» Infection of a bone (osteomyelitis)

HEMOGLOBIN A1C (HBA1C)

The A1c, HbA1c, is "critical in the management of both type 1 and type 2 diabetes", says Fran Kaufman, MD, president of the American Diabetes Association. In the US, type 2 diabetes is diagnosed when hemoglobin A1c levels reach 6.5 percent or higher. The higher A1c levels are, the greater the risk of other health problems. Sometimes the condition can be managed through changes in diet, but other patients with type 2 diabetes may need medication, such as insulin or metformin, to help lower their blood sugar levels, and ultimately, reduce the risk of diabetes. This test is a marker of your average blood sugar over about a three-to four-month period of time. There is also a striking correlation between hemoglobin A1c and the rate at which your brain is shrinking. Both of these factors, your blood sugar and hemoglobin A1c, are entirely within your power to control, as they respond to dietary changes.

IRON

Iron is essential for human life, as it is a key part of various proteins and enzymes involved in the transportation of oxygen and the regulation of cell growth and differentiation, among many other uses. One of the most important roles of iron is to provide hemoglobin (the protein in red blood cells), a mechanism through which it can bind to oxygen and carry it throughout your tissues. Without proper oxygenation, your cells quickly start dying. If you have too little iron, you may experience fatigue, decreased immunity, or iron-deficiency anemia, which can be serious if left untreated. This is common in children and premenopausal women. Checking your iron levels is one of the most important tests that everyone should have done on a regular basis as part of a preventive, proactive health screen; it can be done with a simple blood test called a serum ferritin test; your ferritin level should be between 20 and 80 ng/ml, and 40 to 60 is ideal. If your iron levels are elevated or you have hemochromatosis, donating your blood or obtaining a prescription for therapeutic phlebotomy is one of the best solutions.

FERRITIN

The serum ferritin test measures your stored iron. While your iron levels may be normal, you may still experience fatigue because the body is not using your iron properly. Ferritin is a protein in the body that binds to iron; most of the iron stored in the body is bound to ferritin. Ferritin is found in the liver, spleen, skeletal muscles, and bone marrow. Only a small amount of ferritin is found in the blood. A ferritin blood test is done to the cause of anemia, especially iron deficiency anemia, see if in or too much iron is present, and to see if an iron treatment is working.

VITAMIN B12

Vitamin B12 is essential, meaning it must come from food or supplementation. One-quarter of U.S. adults suffer from low vitamin B12 levels. One of the hallmarks of low B12 is fatigue, which may mean you don't have enough blood oxygen to supply energy. Anxiousness and depression may occur because a B12 shortage also depresses the brain chemical serotonin, a neurotransmitter linked to your brain's pleasure centers and dopamine, the mood regulator registering memory and mood. Unless there's an intervention, low B12 levels may even lead to paranoia, delusions, and hallucinations. Vitamin B12 is helpful for metabolizing folate, carbohydrates, and fat, forming red blood cells, producing adrenal hormones, and is involved in many other functions.

» Produces adrenal hormones

» Metabolizes folate

» Metabolizes fat and carbohydrates

» Forms red blood cells

» Aids in iron absorption

» Helps ensure proper circulation

» Promotes reproductive health

» Aids in digestion

» Supports nervous system function

» Optimizes nerve growth and function

» Testosterone

» Estrogen

» Progesterone

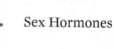 Sex Hormones

- » TSH
- » T3   } Thyroid Hormones
- » T4
- » DHEA   } Adrenal/Stress Hormones
- » Cortisol
- » Vit D
- » CRP
- » A1C
- » Iron
- » Ferritin
- » B12

NATURAL WAYS TO HEAL YOUR HORMONES

While I am a supporter of Bioidentical hormone replacement therapy, I always believe the first place to start is with diet, stress reduction, and lifestyle changes to heal hormones naturally, reducing the need to supplement. To help you remember these five steps of natural hormone health, we are going to use the acronym SHINE.

Sleep - If you want to win the hormone health game, one of the key things is to take a look at how well you sleep. Does it take you longer than 10 or 15 minutes to get to sleep? Do you need to take some kind of medication in order to get to sleep? Our bodies have periods of time where we're highly active and then highly inactive, and our adrenal glands and our sex hormones really love recovery between 11:00pm and 1:00am- the sleep that you get before 11:00pm is very valuable.

Not getting enough sleep does a number of things. One is that it lowers your insulin sensitivity, which means not pulling the sugar out of your bloodstream as effectively. There's a connection between inadequate sleep,weight gain and belly fat. You cannot unlock your body fat if your cortisol levels are too high. We are now finding out that sleep, particularly during the hours of 11pm and 1 o'clock in the morning is specifically important for helping to restore hormones such as sex, thyroid, and adrenals. Going to sleep in deep darkness can help you to get into the stage 4 sleep, which is the deepest, most restorative kind of sleep. Learn the science of sleep and figure out what you can do to improve your sleep without having to use Ambient. Learn about the nutrients that would help to restore sleep and foods that increase melatonin-melatonin being one of the amazing hormones that regulates your sleep/wake rhythms and improves immunity. Sleep is the first factor and most overlooked, the body can optimally repair and replenish much on its own by getting this step under control.

Hormones - A few of the mother hormones, which start off with Pregnenolone and DHEA, are made from cholesterol. We have a cholesterol war that's happening, in which the medical community is really encouraging people to get their cholesterol levels down as low as possible. Unfortunately, this is all being driven by big pharmaceutical companies that are manufacturing cholesterol-lowering medications. Within functional medicine, it's really important that we don't get people's cholesterol levels so low because you don't have the substrates to make your hormones. Functional medicine recommendations are HDL levels above 40, especially for women, LDL levels at 120 or lower and total cholesterol at 220 or lower. Cholesterol is a repair nutrient that repairs blood vessels that have been damaged by toxins that create inflammation, so be extremely cautious when considering medication. Doctors and pharmaceutical companies are politically and financially tied and there are many natural ways to lower cholesterol that have less harmful side effects.

Investigate your stress - Do you feel out of balance or often find that many things cause your heart to race and feel out of control? When we find ourselves getting angry or frustrated, we're creating patterns within the body that are affecting our hormones. It starts with our sympathetic and parasympathetic nervous system. Stress has an impact, and instead of focusing on stress management, I encourage stress reduction and elimination, which will be covered more thoroughly, in Chapter 12.

Nutrition - There's a completely new area in the field of medicine called nutrition endocrinology and it's looking at the impact of what we eat and how food can really help us to reset our hormones. If you're struggling with releasing weight and sense that you have sugar cravings, we can guess that your cortisol levels are possibly higher or the sex hormones are low. In this case, focus on getting more carbohydrates coming from low-starch vegetables and less grains.

For example, we have already talked about gluten. Gluten is a protein found in wheat, rye, and barley, and a good percentage of the population can't metabolize it due to lacking the enzymes to break it down. What happens is it actually causes damage at the villi level of the gut and exposing yourself to a toxin like gluten, over a lifetime, can have an impact on your thyroid. It can cause your thyroid to work harder. Grains in general can drive up cortisol, which can drive up insulin. Cortisol and insulin both have a lot to do with storing body fat, whereas if you restrain the grains and look at how to get more vegetables in, there can be a huge reset. Not only resetting the metabolic hormones, but also stress and sex hormones, and that is a small example of how nutrition effects natural hormone regulation.

Exercise – This can stimulate production of human growth hormone (HGH) every day just by simply triggering the release of growth hormone through strenuous physical activity. No need to work out like a maniac, overtraining will affect the ability to produce human growth hormone. Increase the intensity and resistance during workouts, but include proper rest in between sets and even days of training.

HGH, Human growth hormone, can be synthesized every single night just through proper exercise. Human growth hormone is responsible for so many things, such as improving your muscle mass, immunity, and keeping body fat levels down.

Resistance training is more effective at improving those hormones and your human growth hormone will not even turn on if there is not an adequate amount of sleep.

CHAPTER 12

SECRET 4: EMBRACING & PROCESSING FEELINGS

"The emotion that can break your heart is sometimes the very one that heals it ."

Nicholas Sparks

E MOTION IS ENERGY. The biggest invisible factor for releasing weight and changing behavior is emotion, yet this is the least understood component. In Chapter 3, we talked about healing digestion and uncovering foods that not only cause leaky gut, but also stimulate cravings. The biochemistry of our food can have an emotional impact; sugar can give you a high, as well as a crash that feels like depression. Cleaning up the diet and removing inflammatory foods can eliminate cravings and balance mood and emotions.

Secret 3 was to connect some of the symptoms with hormones that may be depleted or out of balance. Dr. Allen Peters and Dr. Elizabeth Plourde were both prescribed anti-depressants to alleviate their symptoms, but both of these physicians knew it was a hormonal imbalance causing their lack of energy and mood, not depression. Balance the hormones and you may feel calm and vitalized again. Once your biochemistry and neurotransmitters, that control your brain chemistry, are all working optimally, then it will be time to focus on the continued habits and coping mechanisms, like food and alcohol, which come from an emotional trigger.

If we don't learn how to express, release, and then process our emotions, we will be forever susceptible to being triggered and reach for that "thing" that helps us to feel comfort, control, and calm. This is an addiction.

You have at least one addiction, we all do.

Most people think about alcohol and drugs when they hear the word addiction. However, an addiction is any habit or belief that stops us from feeling what is in our hearts. It is anything that keeps us distracted from movement forward in our lives, having what we want, connecting with our true feelings within ourselves, and others. Addictions keep us from our soul's journey of how our life wants to unfold, because it may include painful feelings and uncertainty- this is how we grow and expand.

We are going to start by identifying different kinds and forms of addiction, then how to become more mindful of the behaviors that sabotage healing and true progress. Next, we will break down emotion into a simple process that you can use to move through it, process it, and therefore, eliminate the need to use food, alcohol, or anything else to avoid it. There are two categories of addictions, hard and soft.

HARD ADDICTIONS

» Drugs

» Pain Pills

» Alcohol

» Tobacco

» Food- chips, sugar, carbohydrates

» Coffee

SOFT ADDICTIONS:

» Technology- smart phone, tablet, TV

» Shopping

» Work-a-holism

» Busy-ness

» Need for Control

» Need to look good

» To Do Lists

» Need to be needed

» Need to be right

» Being a Victim

» Aloofness- not being present

» In constant chaos- always putting out fires

The most commonly accepted addictions are drugs and alcohol. The next hard addiction that most people are not even aware of is food. While biochemically sugar can have a similar effect on the brain as cocaine, food is the most widely abused addiction and least addressed. A hard addiction is anything you cannot be without for 24 hours or that causes massive anxiety by not having it/doing it.

While there are brain chemistry elements that contribute to hard addictions, the soft addictions can be even more dangerous.

The danger in soft addictions is that all of these are accepted as normal behavior. What makes them an addiction is the over use of the habit or belief that keeps you from sitting with yourself long enough to feel what is in your heart.

HOW DID I GET THIS ADDICTION?

Addiction comes from protecting our wounds when we don't want to feel pain, anger, or grief; it is an unconscious way of protecting wounds that we have from the past. For example, maybe you wanted a more loving relationship with someone in your past and it didn't work. What we usually do is turn to food or alcohol (those are the two big ones) to fill that void. Addiction comes from a void. Either there's something that we don't want to feel that's happened, or we're afraid of it happening when we don't live in our heart.

We have a choice to live in our head or our hearts, but we can't be in two places at the same time. When we live in our heads, this is one of the ways that addictions are born, because we're listening to the ego. The ego is that critical and negative voice telling us to do things that distract us from our path and our souls. You know when you hear that voice that says, "Oh, don't do that. You're not smart enough. You're not good enough," all of those negativities bring us back to that place within us that bring us down and lead us away from what we came here to do and the soul's path. Addictions cover up deep wounds, fear, and grief for what we didn't have. It's any behavior or thing that keeps us out of our authentic self and true self-expression.

An addiction is also a repetitive use of something (or anything) that takes us away from listening to our subconscious mind.

It doesn't have to be food and alcohol. In fact, for many it's an electronic device. Addiction is a circular movement, in energetic terms, of doing the same thing over and over that keeps us in a loop. Learning how to connect with what is driving the need for distraction from the soul is the answer. The addiction is just a symptom.

We can have an addiction to the beliefs that we have about our past and the perceptions and interpretation of what has happened. These perceptions create some type of a hole inside of us and the hole needs to be filled. What we do is, fill it with the things that keep us stuck so that we're not feeling the hole. For many people, feelings are so scary that the addiction helps us to keep running, moving, going, and doing something, so that we are not sitting with ourselves and actually *feeling*.

One of the biggest addictions is the one we all have to control. We are addicted to control. We didn't feel we had it in our earlier years and we try, consciously or unconsciously, to gain the illusion of control with power over people and situations. In daily activities, that to-do list can create some type of control for all of us. Food addictions have a root in control because sometimes people feel that food is the only thing they can control. Anxiety is an indicator of control issues.

Identifying your addictions brings awareness, which is the first step to healing. Care needs to be taken when there is a hard addiction and a need to come off a substance. However, the deeper work is to get to the wound, release the emotional pain, and then the physical addiction is easier to release. It's the energy of the wound that creates the addiction. If you stop one addiction, let's say you give up drinking but then begin to smoke or smoking becomes more, the energy from the wound, when it is not healed, just moves to another way to suppress the emotion. Until that core emotion is dissolved, resolved, and let go of in the body, there will be addiction energy. If the wound is not healed, the addictive energy is still in the body.

IDENTIFYING THE ADDICTION

Start with the mind-body connection and notice physical symptoms that occur before and during a trigger moments. Notice how you are talking to yourself in the conscious mind. Is there self-judgment? Is there lack of drive? What's going on inside of you? Are you watching too much TV? Are you on an electronic device? Are you using sugar or food? Take a moment and ask yourself, "Is my life the happiest it can be? Is my life the best it can be?" and if the answer is no, ask yourself, "What have I not been willing to look at to bring me those things or move me in that direction?" Then you may start to notice the repetitive behavior, things that may feel normal to you, like chaos, excuses, blame, and overdrive. If you have tension in your body, that's a huge tipoff that something is not right.

Sit in a meditative state and get quiet. Let all the distractions go and do some belly breathing. Then ask yourself, "What is it that I really want?" After you figure out the answer to that question, move on to, "Why don't I have that? Then ask yourself, "How can I accomplish what I want?" whether it's a good relationship or work related. Let your intuition come through and guide you. It's really full of wisdom and is such a great resource inside of each of us.

Whatever your answer is, check yourself during the day and make sure your actions are congruent with what you have been wanting. Make sure you're not using a substance or food to move away from that feeling. Stay present with that, and you will begin to find a pattern that you can begin to work on.

When you identify your addictions, ask yourself, "How does sugar, food, Internet... serve me? What part of me is this serving? Is it the part that's afraid? Is it the part that doesn't want to move forward? Is it the part that's angry? What is it that you don't want to feel, deal with, know about, or be responsible for?" Somewhere in that last question, you will find the answer. Fear is a life-crippler. It drains the life out of what you want, out of joy. Once you move past this, you will feel like a completely different person.

KINDS OF THERAPIES

While I have been a proponent of therapy for many years, I have adjusted my stance on this over the last five years, and it has to do with this addiction conversation. In my experience, many therapeutic tools are about managing emotions after being triggered or making plans to avoid being triggered- this is not healing. Traditional talk therapy, which only involves 12% of the conscious mind, is not powerful enough to reprogram the 88% of the subconscious mind and shift that trauma point of origin.

This is why you or someone you know may have been in therapy for years yet they still struggle with similar issues- they haven't healed the root. They may understand it now but the emotional energy is still there. When that core belief and emotional energy exists, it will manifest in different ways. Over the years, I have benefitted from attending certain support groups, like Al-Anon, whose core message elevated and expanded my understanding of the social effects of addiction. However, because everyone is so focused on the addictive behavior, the underlying root and feelings are overlooked. A food addiction is no different, energetically, than cocaine or alcohol. Many times, someone who is a recovering addict of alcohol or tobacco expresses their addiction energy in many other soft addictions like control, technology or food. The addiction energy has not been healed because you stopped (or changed) the addiction habit.

Two therapies I have experienced and recommend for others are hypnosis and EMDR (Eye Movement Desensitizing Reestablishment). Hypnosis can get into the 88% of the subconscious mind and start to change the recording. While there are many programs you can do on your own, I think it is most effective to work with someone privately who can record a personalized hypnosis with your emotional history in mind. EMDR needs to be done with a therapist as well, and can be delivered through ear phones, hand held sensors, or with no equipment, just the therapist's fingers drawing a pattern for your eyes to follow once you land on the emotion. I prefer this last way the best because I have found it to be the fastest and easiest way to get to the emotion in a conscious state. While I am not a licensed therapist, I have healed issues using these techniques.

How do you know when you have healed? You are different in the same situation. The emotions and thoughts that used to be triggered are triggered no more. In place of fear, pain and anxiety is peace, calm, and understanding a clear perspective of what is really happening for the other person. This is called being the observer. When you take something personally, you have been triggered, which means you have something to heal because it's never really about you.

CHAPTER 13

THE ANATOMY OF EMOTION

"The more accurately you can name an emotion,
the quicker you can move through it ."

Brené Brown

L IKE USING THE PHYSICAL sciences of the body to customize workout plans and diets, I love using the psychological sciences to break down thoughts, emotions, and beliefs to problem solve anything and everything. Once you truly understand the anatomy of emotion, I believe you can heal anything.

Most people can identify when they have a strong feeling. The problem is that it is then customary to blame the person or event that you perceive caused the feeling. It is easy to point the finger and say, "Now I am mad so it must be your fault".

This is absolutely incorrect. No one outside of you can **make** you feel anything, ever.

Yet, the majority of us have perpetuated this victim behavior because we have never really had a need to study emotions as we do now. Think about it, what did your parents or grandparents focus on- survival. Putting food on the table and keeping a roof over your head. Who had time to focus on whether or not they were actually happy?

Consciousness and mindfulness is a rather new movement in the last 30-40 years because we are at an abundant time in history where we have time to ask these internal questions of whether or not we are happy. The rate of suicide has been increasing and I believe it is because we have not been given the tools to understand, process, and problem solve emotions.

Everything we choose in life is because we want to feel something- love, relief, safety, acceptance, or anything else. Yet, do you understand how and why you react the way you do to things? Doesn't it seem strange that in certain situations that drive you crazy, other people don't seem bothered? How often do you ask yourself, "What caused me to feel or react this way?" It's time to transform victim behavior because it is the root that keeps addiction energy stuck in your body.

THE BREAKDOWN

Feelings do not just happen. They are a result of a thought and interpretation, whether it is conscious or subconscious. First, we observe or think something next, we interpret it. Based on what we **think** about the situation and what **it means** to us, we then have a **feeling.** Two people can be looking at the same situation and interpret it very differently. What it means to them will determine how they **feel** about it. There is no one "right" way to interpret anything. All negative emotion happens when we feel or perceive a need that is not being met.

Recently when working with a client who often emotionally overeats in the form of binging, I used this system to help her identify what was causing her pain and anxiety. Once we did this process, she had learned a new tool that actually solved the problem at hand instead of turning to food to numb the feelings of anxiety that came up when she focused on it. Not only did she feel relief that she has several options to solve the issue, she felt so empowered that her emotional eating has drastically reduced.

We have to start off with acknowledging what you have power over and what you can control. Other people are walking around with their own wounds and story, so while you may think someone else can cause you pain, they can only reflect back to you what needs to be healed inside of you. The only things you have power over and can control are YOUR thoughts, beliefs, interpretations, feelings, and reactions.

Emotion is energy and once you have been triggered, I first want to encourage you to allow yourself a safe space to feel the emotion. It's not easy to problem solve something when you are caught in the wave of energy that is the emotion. Jumping too quickly to figure it out can also suppress that energy inside your body, which we don't want because negative emotional build up will perpetuate addictions and lead to physical disease.

Please do not skip the feeling part. Emotions are like the weather, they may turn into a tornado or earthquake, but they will pass once the energy is released. Then move onto the three-step process to problem solving so you can get the need met and resolve the issue. **Non Violent Communication**, by Dr. Marshall Rosenberg, breaks this down into simple and usable tools.

1. Identify the emotion(s).
2. Identify the need(s).
3. Create at least one strategy of getting those needs met *that do not require anyone else to do or be different.*

The most important, yet simple, tools is the Feelings and Needs List. Download a copy of it at www.invisiblefitness.com and print many copies. Put one in every room, every bag or briefcase and even in your car. Use it daily to strengthen your emotional IQ and create awareness. Have it handy in the cases where you are feeling negative emotions so you can transform the situation quickly before it accelerates.

FEELINGS AND NEEDS LIST

Step 1 is to identify the feeling(s). When I work with people on identifying emotion, most have an extremely limited vocabulary about their emotional range. Circle all the emotions in the moment, and then focus on the strongest one or two.

FEELINGS

PEACEFUL	PLAYFUL	MAD	CONFUSED	SAD
absorbed	alive	aggravated	apathetic	despair
blissful	effervescent	agitated	embarrassed	despondent
calm	energetic	angry	hesitant	discouraged
content	exuberant	annoyed	perplexed	distressed
engrossed	impish	bitter	torn	gloomy
expansive	invigorated	enraged	troubled	grief
serene	refreshed	exasperated	uncomfortable	heavy
spacious	stimulated	frustrated	uneasy	hopeless
tranquil	zestful	furious	withdrawn	hurt
		hostile		lonely
GLAD	**LOVING**	irritated		pessimistic
confident	affectionate	miffed	**SCARED**	troubled
delighted	appreciative		afraid	vulnerable
encouraged	compassionate	**TIRED**	anxious	
excited	friendly	exhausted	fearful	
grateful	nurtured/nurturing	fatigued	horrified	
happy	sensitive	fidgety	jittery	
hopeful	tender	indifferent	nervous	
inspired	warm	lethargic	panicky	
joyful	sweet	listless	shocked	
relieved		overwhelmed	startled	
satisfied		weary	terrified	
			worried	

Step 2 is to identify the need(s) that is not being met for you, not someone else. Avoid saying, "I need him to.." or " My need is for her to...". The need you are uncovering is yours in general, not in relationship to any specific person, thing, or situation. This is probably the most difficult step because we have not been taught to be aware of even having needs, let alone getting them met.

NEEDS

MEANING	AUTONOMY	CONNECTION	PHYSICAL	COMMUNITY
Acknowledgment	Choice	Acceptance	Air	Collaboration
Awareness	Freedom	Belonging	Hydration	Cooperation
Beauty	Independence	Closeness	Movement	Equality
Celebration	Space	Communication	Procreation	Inclusion
Clarity		Companionship	Rest	Mutuality
Closure	**AUTHENTICITY**	Compassion	Safety	Support
Competence	Aliveness	Consideration	Shelter	
Contribution	Creativity	Empathy	Sustenance	**PEACE**
Effectiveness	Honesty	Interdependence	Touch	Beauty
Growth	Integrity	Intimacy		Conciousness
Hope	Openess	Love	**PLAY**	Ease
Inspiration	Self Expression	Respect	Excitement	Flow
Learning	To be heard/seen	Sexual Expression	Fun	Harmony
Mourning	To know/be known		Humour	Presence
Mystery	Transparency		Joy	Spaciousness
Purpose	Trust		Laughter	Spiritual
Connection				
Stimulation				Transformation
Understanding				

Emotional manipulation, especially from women to men and parents to children, is often because the manipulator has a need that they believe someone else is responsible for. Parents manipulate their children into behavior that is pleasing to the parent at the expense of the child. A child might be enjoying an activity that creates fear in a parent so the parent demands the child change so they can feel more at ease while the child learns that they can ask others to behave differently until it pleases them. It's a viscous cycle that not only doesn't work and leads to addiction, but isn't even logical. No one is happy when they are asked to deny their own feelings for someone else. Happiness is an inside job and no one is required to behave in ways that please you first. If we could all get this right, there would be many happier people with less depression, war, and fighting. This step might also create awareness of major changes that need to be made in your life. Once you take responsibility for your needs and feelings, how you interpret situations in your life may change.

Step 3 becomes easier when you realize that the need you have has to be met by you first. Creating multiple strategies help you to see that you are not a victim to circumstance and that you can create a win-win situation with most people. Everyone is selfishly only able to ask for what they need first, and if they aren't asking for help, they will use emotional manipulation to get the need met consciously or subconsciously. There will be relief the minute you create a few strategies to get your need met. Once you see the power you have over your life to change how you feel, these steps will get easier and easier. Empowerment feels good and can bring you peace. Victim mentality will keep you stuck and powerless.

To outline these steps in action, I will give you a personal example. Whenever I have a negative feeling that won't let up, I use the Feelings and Need list and do this process.

My husband and I were scheduled to go to a weekend event that evoked negative feelings in me every time I thought about it. He told me I didn't have to go, but I wanted to support him, so I made a point to work through my feelings and transform it into something that could feel better to me.

First, I observed my physical response to the idea- my body caved in, my shoulders rounded forward and I felt a pit in my stomach. Next, I explored what my feelings were; I was feeling trapped, a lack of freedom, and worry. What needs of mine were not being met? The answer was my need for freedom (in a few areas) and connection.

Next, I asked myself, what I could do to provide myself the freedom I needed in this situation and then I provided that for myself. I did the same with connection- I gave myself permission to connect with myself first and then be open to connecting with others but not to be dependent on or expect to get it from anyone else. Because I made sure to have a solution for each need, not only did I feel better but I also had a better time. I attracted more connection from others because I was already at peace within myself.

HOW EMOTIONS CREATE DISEASE

Disease and illness can start as thoughts. If you think thoughts such as, "Oh, I'm never going to get this job, I'm never going to find a relationship," which are negative thoughts that come from the ego (the critical voice), the body absorbs that energy. The organs and tissues of the body take in that stress, which over time will cause break down.

We accept that when we feel embarrassed, the face turns red. When you feel nervous, there are "butterflies" or a "pit" in your stomach. When you get startled, the heart beats faster. When you have negative, toxic emotions, where do you think that goes? The difference between how we behave is based on what's inside of us. For example, compare someone who handles traffic well and someone who gets really angry. The angry person might increase blood pressure. Why is it different for these two people? It goes back to an emotional feeling that maybe they were trapped as a kid. Maybe they didn't like their family environment. Maybe it was hostile or unsafe. Sitting in traffic recreates the feeling of being trapped. The traffic is the 10% that triggers that 90% of stuck emotional memory in our subconscious but most people are unaware of it.

Most people are not aware of the impact of old memories-feelings buried alive do not die. This is also what is considered a trauma. Many people think, "Oh, I don't have any traumas.", but we all do. That just means you're not aware of them as traumas, but your body recognizes them as traumas. Think of a walnut and the wounds is in the center. We build these protective coatings around us like the shell of the walnut so people can't get close to us because we're afraid of being hurt-we're protecting the wound. If you don't have what you want or you're not happy in any area of your life, there's something blocking it. It may be a trauma or a well-established pattern. We establish these protective layers so that people can't get to us.

Anxiety is not really a feeling; it's a body sensation, letting us know that there are unresolved feelings. It's a vibration that says there's something that wants to come out. When you work with the true feelings, (grief, sadness, pain, and anger) whatever feeling is underneath that anxiety, the anxiety can then be released and goes away. Anxiety is a message. If you're worrying about something or feel anxious, there's something underneath that, which needs to be released. When buried alive, they still have their own vibration and can cause disharmony in our systems.

The feeling of unsafe can go into shoulder pain, back pain, or headaches. Respiratory things can also occur because people stop breathing correctly when there is anxiety present. Fatigue can occur as well because we're using the energy to keep the anxiety alive as we keep feeding it.

Emotional pain is in there, and it's running your life. You don't even know it. You're making decisions based on fear. For instance, people take a safe job rather than go out into the world and do what they want. They choose safe relationships, which maybe you don't get to be in your power. Maybe you don't feel empowered in the relationship. Maybe it's just playing it safe. Therefore, I ask you, "Are you okay to live the way you're living, or would you rather take your chance and dip your toe in the pool and see what the pool feels like?"

Listen to your body. Whenever you feel a charge in your body, a movement, energy, clenching, or pain, the body is your best barometer to what's going on. Next, notice if you are reacting from a place of what you need or if you are just reacting to what somebody is doing or saying. Ninety percent of most folks live in reaction to life, rather than grabbing it by the horns and taking it where they want it to go and allowing it to go.

Let your body be the guide- pain is a message. As you experience a physical pain or something inside of you, stop, be aware of it, and take a few breaths. Sit with yourself, and ask, "What is this about?" Empty your mind as best as you can, because you want to move away from the critical voice that has begun the process of creating the physical pain, or the body sensation that you're having, like anxiety. You can't have anxiety unless it's connecting to something inside. When you get to a calm place, ask your body, "What are you trying to tell me?" Sit and wait for the answer. If you don't get the answer, it usually means that your head is still going. You're not fully engaged with your solar plexus, your breathing. My favorite resource that can help uncover the emotional root to physical pain and disease is ***Messages from The Body,*** Michael J Lincoln, Ph.D.

CHAPTER 14

HOW TO STOP SHAMING YOURSELF

"Shame corrodes the very part of us that believes
we are capable of change ."

Brené Brown

IT ALL STARTS WITH the self-talk in your head. There is a word we use in judging others and ourselves that inflicts violence and we are not even aware of it. It's one little word that most of us use all the time-- **should.**

Marshall Rosenberg, author and founder of **Nonviolent Communication**, teaches that the word "should" is the most violent word we use because it indicates that we do not have a choice. Brené Brown, author of **Gifts of Imperfection** and **Daring Greatly**, would probably say that "should" is shaming and I'd agree. Freedom is one of the most important concepts I live by, teach with, and offer others so this concept is huge for me.

After learning this, I started to notice how many times I use that word, both for my clients and me. Wow! It is not my intention to shame or lock anyone into something they are not choosing–ever!

A few months ago, I was doing the dishes, pissed off because a so-called friend bailed, yet again, from a function, and I had been torn about what to do about it. As the water was running, I told myself, "***You should just leave it be and allow it. You can't control it.***" and then I immediately stopped and froze. I just told myself I "should"!

Should feels like "trapped" to me- no freedom and no choice. My body tightens, my heart sinks, my stomach clenches, and the anger starts to bubble up inside of me.

While I do not have a choice about how someone else behaves, communicates, interprets, or even feels, I do have complete choice about how I respond to it. I started by acknowledging how I felt.

You may think because I am a trainer and coach, that I "should" guilt my clients about food or exercise, but I don't. One of my clients years ago told me that she chose me because I "allowed" her to have her ice cream. These were her words, I would never pretend to take power away from someone's choice or shame/guilt them with my desires for them. I was actually branded America's Guilt Free Trainer for a while because I empower my clients, not treat them like naughty children!

This little word permeates the fitness and health industry like a lurking big brother or mother who is going to punish you if you don't do as you **should**. It's no wonder why people say they lack motivation!

When you set yourself up like that and do not complete or follow through, you diminish the confidence in yourself. You are actually shaming yourself with this one little word. I know I have done it too. It's why I rebel against the industry standard of either looking like a bodybuilder or a twig.

Accepting myself for who I am, where I am, and what I want is the first step to self-respect and the place where I have found success in all areas of life. **Should**-ing is disrespecting and disempowering and comes from a place of fear, not love.

What do you want, and why do you want it? Drown out the **shoulds**- they do not motivate you long term, and they threaten the respect and trust you have in yourself. Replace **should** with **want**; see how you respond differently, especially with food, exercise, and self-care.

EXERCISE AS THERAPY

Over the last twenty years, I have not only used exercise to soothe my mood but to unlock and release stuck emotional energy. Movement can be a powerful tool for emotional release as well as releasing weight, increasing strength, flexibility, longevity, and general health- exercise can become therapy! When you use exercise as a therapeutic tool, you transform the act of exercising into a form of love, which can heal body shame.

A placebo-controlled study conducted by James Blumenthal, professor of psychology at Duke University, was published in an issue of the journal *Psychosomatic Medicine*. The study compared exercise to a common antidepressant medication in a group of individuals diagnosed with major depressive disorder, and found that *exercise was as effective as the drug* at alleviating symptoms of the disorder. Exercise is clinically more effective than drugs to elevate your mood because emotion is energy.

Before my husband and I met, I had an argument with a guy I was dating. Frustrated and angry, I could feel that displeasure well up inside of me like a fireball that needed a target. Due to the inconvenient fact that I was volunteering at a workshop for the weekend, I didn't have any time to go to the gym or even step outside for more than ten minutes. Assessing my need to hit something, I took a friend to the bathroom, grabbed the seat cushion from the lounge chair, handed it to her, and said, "Can you hold this? I am going to kick and punch it."

Within three strikes, the third one including a loud grunt of frustration, the bubble of emotion inside of me had been broken and tears were streaming down my face. Without too many words, I acknowledged my anger, which was really masking the fear of being rejected, and then felt a sigh of great relief. Once I could identify it and release it, it no longer had power over me. I was free! My energy level came back to normal and I was the happy, pleasant person I normally am, and I felt clear-headed and calm all within five minutes.

Emotions sometimes create a barrier and add resistance to you moving forward, so choosing the appropriate exercise can make all the difference in soothing or releasing what you might be going through. There are many different types of exercises out there and I will be not able to cover them all but here are a few to start with and try out in your own routines.

Anger has energy to it, the frequency and intensity of thoughts that are going on in your mind and transmitting to your body need to find a release in order for the anger to move through you. Kickboxing, boxing, and running are great ways to give your body an outlet for these emotions. The impact of your body against the ground, a heavy bag, or some focus mitts can help release that tension (and adding sound is even more effective!) Sexual frustrations can also be eased with these same exercises.

Anxiety has energy to it as well but less streamlined than anger. If anger is focused tension, anxiety is nervous energy that is unfocused and all over the place. Because you are unfocused, organizing your thoughts to the present moment will help calm you down. Using mindful resistance training, which means focusing on what is going on in the body and recruiting muscle fibers with your mind, and high impact cardio classes bring you into the present moment. Efficient resistance training requires that you be in tune with your body and using your brainpower to engage your muscles. If your mind is somewhere else, not only are you not getting the optimal benefits from the exercise, you could injure yourself, because you are not in tune with the body's messages of when you are nearing failure and fatigue. Choreographed cardio classes will also require that you are in the moment and provide an opportunity for you to focus so you can ignore the worry about the future or replaying something from the past in your mind.

Sadness, depression, and fear are emotions that have less or blocked energy. Ease of movement is the most important factor in dealing with this low-level status, so walking would be my first recommendation. Most of us walk for some duration of time in a day, even if it's around the house; increasing the duration interrupts the pattern of thought and you start to think about different things. Rollerblading or biking provides a gliding that the body doesn't do without wheels. The momentum of energy created from the wheels is an instant pick me up - you are using less energy while the ease of gliding is comforting. Dancing is also a great way to combat sadness, depression, and fear because of the power of music. Choose a dance that is appropriate for music you like or a dance that feels good in your body. Take a few classes in different kinds of dance to find the one that really inspires you - it's a great workout too!

Adrenal fatigue and burn out require a different kind of restorative energy; fast paced or high intensity movement will only challenge the body to heal itself even more. Isometric training, hatha yoga, and Pilates would be best in combating burnout. Start by asking yourself how it is you feel, and what you might need to feel better. Rather than skipping the workout because you are cranky, use your exercise to move through that. You'll get your workout in and feel better when it's done!

CHAPTER 15

SECRET 5: THE COURAGE TO CONNECT

"We are here to awaken from the illusion of our separateness."

Thich Nhat Hanh

I T TAKES COURAGE to be vulnerable when we want to connect with other people, but it also takes courage to be honest and connect with ourselves. Something that I don't talk about often or try to affirm is how different I have felt my whole life, even today. As I sit and write this book, I find myself editing how to say what I want to in a way that more people can hear. Fear of being judged, failing, being wrong, or rejected comes up for me more than you might guess. However, because I know that this work is powerful in helping people to make real change and experience healing in their lives, I keep going, because I believe that is why I am here.

We all have a story that keeps us from taking risks. "What if I fail?", "What if I succeed?", and "What if I do nothing?" Researcher and author Brené Brown says that the biggest pain people experience is the pain of being on the sidelines. People who wonder, "What would have happened if I had just shown up and been seen?" In order to release weight and end body shame, we have to be willing to be seen and heard. We also have to be willing to love ourselves in a way that we never have before. Lastly, we need to recognize that our impulse to judge another is really just us rejecting ourselves, and it's mirror to show us what needs to be accepted within us.

This takes courage and support- who supports **your** growth? Because we all have a need to belong and feel "normal", the tribe you have around you might subconsciously sabotage you in order to keep the status quo. When one person expands to make change, it often triggers unhealed wounds in others that cause them to feel uncomfortable. "Who do you think you are?", "What makes you so special?", "How selfish of you?" are phrases I have had directed at me from relatives or people in my past as I was starting my business or making choices that triggered them. There is nothing like being rejected by close family and friends who you thought were there to support your happiness and success. Tribal rejection is a very deep wound. Breaking the patterns of "normal" creates discomfort in those around you, which is why many people really don't dare to be vulnerable and believe in themselves.

Shame and blame are hard to come out from under when all we want is to be loved and accepted. However, as we covered in Chapter 12, everything starts with how we get our own needs met first. We can't give to others what we don't have.

In Brené Brown's second book, *Gifts of Imperfection: Let Go of Who You Think You're Supposed to Be and Embrace Who You Are*, she shares research on what attributes to cultivate to live a "wholehearted life" as well as habits to let go of that keep us safe, but in pain and longing. Take a look at this list and assess which traits reflect your current choices and where you would like to experience change.

CULTIVATE	LET GO
Authenticity	Of What Other's Think of You
Self-Compassion	Perfectionism
Resilient Spirit	Numbing with Addictions
Gratitude & Joy	Scarcity & Fear of the Dark
Intuition & Trust	Need for Certainty (control
Creativity	Comparing Yourself to Others
Play & Rest	Exhaustion as Status Symbol
Calm & Stillness	Anxiety as a Lifestyle
Meaningful Work	Self-Doubt and "Supposed to"
Laughter, Song & Dance	Being cool & in control

How many of these created a painful new awareness for you? In Chapter 12, we uncovered that everything in the list to "let go" of, is really an addiction. Reading a book can bring attention and a new consciousness to our behavior, but how do you make real change? It is easy to give lip service to healing and change while we comfortably stay in our patterns, unwilling to be vulnerable and ask for help. We surround ourselves with people who tell us what we want to hear because of a deep wound that we are not enough, so we keep choosing people who validate everything we do. While it feels good to be accepted, our patterns never heal without the courage to make real change.

Asking for help has been stigmatized as weakness or triggers the "I am not smart enough" or " I am not good enough" belief in people. We keep this illusion alive, refusing to ask for help and then cycling through the patterns of addiction and denial until some big health or life scare occurs. I find it slightly amusing that the people in our lives who have modeled and taught us that asking for help equals weakness are usually the most unhappy, unhealthy, and least self-expressed people. *"**You are the average of the five people you spend the most time with**."* Jim Rohn. Does your tribe support your growth and healing?

We need support and people in our lives who will allow us to try new things and ways of being without judging us. Most people that struggle with releasing weight are great caregivers to other but not to themselves. Why is it that we respect that caregiving quality within ourselves, but are unwilling to give someone else that chance to be that in return for us? In order for someone to be a giver, there has to be a receiver. It's 50/50 and both parts have to exist for there to be an exchange. There is a reason you are not allowing yourself to receive.

RADICAL SELF-FORGIVENESS

Another great resource for healing that I recommend is, Colin Tipping's ***Radical Self Forgiveness: Tools for Achieving Self-Acceptance.*** There is an audio exercise and worksheet in the program that helps to identify areas where you need to forgive yourself and accept that the situation has lessons or reasons beyond your comprehension. One of the reasons we stop ourselves from growing or becoming is that we are often punishing ourselves for something we think we did wrong. Maybe someone told you that what you did was wrong or it was your interpretation. Religion or cultural beliefs may support self-punishment as a form of respect or reverence. Identifying the root of what stops you from fully stepping into who you want to be, is how to start healing it.

Next, just as we covered in Chapter 12, there will be a need to release it energetically in the form of feelings. I recommend Colin Tipping's full audio program in order to get the powerful audio exercise for the greatest impact, I also want to start the process off for you now. On a separate piece of paper, or in a journal, complete these sentences and write whatever comes up for you. If you are fully committed to this exercise, write each phrase on a separate page and allow yourself to bounce around, when the flow stops with one feeling, move to another.

» I blame myself for....

» I feel guilty because...

» I feel anger because...

» I feel shame because...

» I feel sad because...

Take your time with this, allow any and all feelings to come up. After you feel "emptied" and "complete" with expressing all emotional energy from this, ask yourself, "What has been the payoff for holding onto these feelings?"

For example, when I first did the exercise, many years ago, the strongest emotion that came up for me was guilt. I felt sad and guilty that I was not going home more to visit my parents, because I missed them. I had journaled and cried hard for what seemed like hours (it was only minutes), over how badly I felt, and what a terrible daughter I was for not going home. Then the question was asked, "What was the payoff?" Boy did that hit me like a brick! Shocked, I realized that by holding onto the guilt, I was punishing myself so therefore, I didn't have to go home! As long as I felt badly about it, I could keep NOT doing it and feel justified. The truth was I didn't want to go home. While I missed my parents, I wanted them to visit me. I really didn't want to go back "home". The truth felt harsh to admit- what kind of person am I that I didn't want to go home to where I grew up? My own judgement and unwillingness to accept that my feelings were valid and the thought that it was okay to want what I wanted kept me stuck in an emotional pattern that not only affected my business but my health. So let me ask you again, what is the payoff for holding onto these feelings and blame?

Once you have that "aha" moment, ask yourself these questions included in Colin Tipping's **Radical Self Forgiveness**:

» Even if you don't understand how or why, are you willing to be open to the possibility that the situation has been created for your spiritual growth?

» Are you willing to give up your need to judge yourself and your action as right or wrong, good or bad?

» Can you be open to the idea that all that you have done or are doing currently is totally purposeful in the grand scheme of things? And that what you judge about yourself might be exactly what is called for in the divine plan and that you could be a healing angel for someone?

» Are you willing to be open to the idea that you attracted them into your life so you can reconnect to your true nature and access the power within you?

If you answered yes to all of them, we can move on. Often healing and self-forgiveness is about expanding our perception and awareness beyond which we can understand or prove. That's where faith and trust comes into play; the illusion of control often needs a reality check. We live in our little boxes (houses) in our little bubble and forget there is a universe bigger than we can imagine. Most of the stories that we tell ourselves have been created by us out of patterns that keep us stuck and lack truth and accuracy. How often do you tell yourself a story where you play all the parts, deciding for everyone else how they would react or answer and then come out of your head and bring that energy into your reality? Those stories create emotional and mental momentum. In fact, we are always creating some kind of momentum of either allowing or resisting, as well as positive or negative energy.

MOMENTUM

Momentum is happening every day in your life. The question to answer, is that momentum positive and forward moving or negatively reinforcing limited beliefs and habits keeping you stuck and repeating patterns? Albert Einstein said, *"You can't solve a problem with the same mind that created it."* When it comes to healing old wounds, creating new patterns, and making real change in our lives, it's insanity to believe that people could do it by themselves. Can you learn new things? Of course, someone will have to teach it to you since it's not something you have thought before or experienced.

Thoughts are the first place that momentum starts. From the moment we wake up in the morning, the monkey mind starts going unless we train ourselves into a new frequency. I have an online 30-Day Manifestation Challenge that I run and one of the recommendations I make, to shift momentum quickly, is to do a guided visualization. In the program, I created a chakra clearing audio, as well as an imaged focused visualization to use with a vision board. Both are designed to have you focus on your breath first, and then move into connecting with your body. Many of us need to be grounded before we can move into a new frequency of being. Other ways to start changing those thoughts are replacing them with affirmations. Affirmations can be created for every reason: money, love, health, and healing. Doing them often helps to retrain and reprogram thoughts and responses. When you can elevate your frequency and vibration from fear to hopeful, you allow yourself to connect with the energy that is hopeful, allowing you to attract at that level.

Our default mode is often negative. We have been trained to focus on what is not working, what we don't have, and why we don't have it. Imagine you are holding two hand weights- one is 1lb and the other is 10lbs. It is easier to lift the 1lb weight, so you may practice and enforce that more often because it's easier. The 10lbs will make you stronger, but will be more work and much harder. When we do not deliberately focus our thoughts and attention, we default to what is easier and habitual. The good news is that when you practice lifting the 10lbs more often, it also becomes easier in time. Training your focus, point of attraction, thoughts and feelings is no different than training the body. You get good at what you practice.

FIND YOUR TRIBE

Until I started working with the Feelings & Needs list, I couldn't articulate that what I needed was community. Once I figured that out, it felt easier to identify how important community is for people. It's why many people go to church! Ethnic groups, religious groups, neighborhoods, sports teams, social dance groups, PTA, and all common interest groups provide support and education on specific areas of life.

For every new business venture I have started, I joined a group to learn, be accountable, and participate in a community that was focused on the same goals. When times are tough, there are people to help you. Success stories of overcoming obstacles would appear at just the right time to infuse a renewed hope and keep me going. Going at it alone makes it hard to have perspective about the progress being made, and it is a lot easier to quit when no one else is looking. ***"One of the most important things you can do on this earth is to let people know they are not alone"*** Shannon L. Alder, author of ***300 Questions to Ask Your Parents Before It's Too Late***

My clients have many success stories but I wanted to feature one in particular that embodies many of the principles covered in this book. I want to introduce you to one of my clients, Maureen.

I started my journey to adopt a healthier lifestyle over five years ago. At first, all I tried to do was be mindful trying to tune in to see when I was starting to feel full. Once I felt comfortable with that, I started making changes in what I ate and how much. I took small steps because I knew that if I tried to do too much too soon, I would become discouraged.

When I did add exercise to my routine, I first had to become accountable. I promised that I would go to the health club on my 2 days off per week. I think in this whole process for me being accountable is the key. I would also ask myself if eating something or not going to exercise was "in line with my goals".

Before I met with you, I thought I needed to add more days to my exercise routine. You showed me through FITT that I could still accomplish my goals by exercising 2X/week. By changing the intensity and/or type, I would continue to challenge my body/ mind for change.

Since I started this journey, working with you and Dr. Lisa Galper, I have lost a total of 100lbs.

I do believe that things do happen for a reason. Motivation to change has to start from within. For lasting change in habits/ behaviors, I believe you have to be a bit selfish. I am grateful for the knowledge and support that you and Dr. Lisa have provided.

I also learned a lot in your cooking classes. When I do take time to cook, it always seems to be an involved recipe. I learned that I can cook and enjoy things that are much easier to make.

I've been thinking a lot lately about what has lead to my total successes and I think it's being willing to be vulnerable. Here is what I have come up with for me:

» *Walking through the door the first time not knowing what is on the other side*

» *Not knowing that what is on the other side of the door is exactly what you needed.*

» *Realizing that you need to learn, grow, and listen.*

» *Being open to changing habits.*

» *Remembering to keep opening new doors and trying new things.*

» *Having fear and still going for it*

» *Showing up and being seen*

» *Sharing*

Because of my exercise program, I can have more active in life. I used to dread coming home from a long day as that meant I had to walk up a flight of stairs. Now I can run up them. I look forward to the days when I can go do a workout. I find that I miss it when I can't get there. I can look forward to hiking up Masada this spring instead of taking the tram up. I'm grateful that when I decided to open doors, you and Dr. Lisa were on the other side. Many people have tried to show me what you have and failed. My success is based on the fact that I chose to walk through doors, I continue to be receptive to what you have to teach me, and I have created accountability with you and Dr. Lisa this entire time. I think successful, long lasting weight loss has to include dealing with all aspects of life... both physical (exercise and diet) and emotional (or the importance of why). I trust the process that even on the days that I struggle, the support I have is always there. The skills I have developed with JJ's guidance are always there.

I share Maureen's story for a few reasons:

» Healing and change take time

» Healing and change take support

» We created and adjusted a workout that kept giving results for many years; only working out twice a week, and not the 5-7 days that most people assume they need for major change

» Maureen released 100lbs because of a lifestyle change over time, not a quick fix diet

» Maureen is a part of several tribes, including mine, that keeps her accountable and connected to others on a similar journey

» She is working with the whole package- physical, emotional, and spiritual

"You will never change your life until you change something you do daily . The secret of your success is found in your daily routine ."

John C Maxwell, author of *No Limits*

I would love to support you on this journey. If you are interested in learning more, please visit ***invisiblefitnessacademy. com***

WHAT PEOPLE ARE SAYING

"Before JJ, I was regularly working out in my garage on my equipment getting nowhere. I have always been active and exercised, so I thought I knew what I was doing. I also had knee pain, back pain and a few pounds to lose. It's now been 8 years and I have not only worked with JJ over the phone and one on one in person, I even hired her to create a Wellness Program for my company. My knee pain was alleviated within the first few months, I released 10 lbs easily after going gluten and dairy free and I feel stronger and faster on the ski slopes than I have in years. JJ Flizanes is not only my trainer, she is my confident, shrink, strategist, nutritionist and counselor. Her knowledge and wisdom goes beyond the sciences of the body. And I wouldn't trust my joints to anyone else- I need them to keep up with my active lifestyle."

Jody Lay

"JJ is the most holistic trainer/coach I have ever worked with. Although I view her specialty as being in the areas of exercise and diet, she has the gift of seeing ALL areas of my life and how they work together to support or sabotage me. JJ takes my lifestyle into consideration rather than trying to change my lifestyle to fit her philosophy. This has been my experience a lot in the past with other trainers/nutritionists. And did I stick with them...NOPE. Because JJ has the ability to work with my lifestyle starting where I'm at, she is the only trainer that I have returned to over and over for tune-ups over the years. I never feel judged by her. I feel accepted RIGHT WHERE I'M AT when in her presence and we always start from there and that's the biggest gift to me. Sometimes it's hard for even me to accept myself where I'm at. So, she takes the first step and I follow.

JJ has a unique balance of nudging me to live a healthier lifestyle without having me feel judged. I don't know how she does it but this is one of her many gifts that I experience in each communication with her. JJ supported me in losing 35 pounds and assisted me in bringing light into the blind spots that I had not seen for many years. She is a true motivator that is committed to her clients I used to use a scale to measure how I was doing with my health and fitness goals. In working with JJ, she helped me to uncover that I had my self-worth tied to this number so out the scale went! She also helped me to see how I was repeatedly shaming myself when the number was not a good enough or an acceptable number. She then taught me how that shame kept me locked in a vicious cycle that kept me stuck for many years. JJ is all about accepting you right where you are and starting from there through compassion and loving empowerment!"

Audre Nelson, LMFT

"Wow! Wow! Wow! A one-stop book!

JJ has woven multiple disciplines to create a masterpiece! There is not another book out there that combines all of these essential principals.

Well-being is not just about how one looks through diet and exercise. It about what we feel inside. JJ has it right... emotion IS energy. If our internal emotions are not 'clean' meaning that someone has not fully processed and released emotions, then there is a high probability of addiction. JJ's examples of addictions will surprise you but she is right.

JJ has given us all the tools under one cover! If you want to change your life, take the time to read this extraordinary book and follow JJ's guidance."

Pam Knight

"Since our first session I lost more than 25 pounds, lost two pants sizes and gained strength as well as flexibility. There is no doubt that I could not have achieved the weight loss without JJ's innovative and ever changing exercise program. JJ's routines are highly effective as well as being sensitive not to aggravate old injuries. Consequently, I had the gain with no pain. On top of being extremely knowledgeable in the field of physical fitness, she also has a great personality. She knows how to motivate and encourage moving on to ever more advanced routines. I found her next-day follow ups to be very helpful in judging how effective the workout was. Put all this together, assures me that I am in very good hands indeed. In short, she is a keeper. "

Dr. Michael Schapa

"We first met JJ at a demonstration workshop and immediately hired her to work with me. I needed help strengthening my back which had issues due to a severe in-flight air-turbulence injury acquired long ago. As the primary caregiver for my severely handicapped mother, lifting wheelchairs in and out of cars and holding up and onto mom as she transferred to or from them, I was at constant risk of re-injury. JJ is amazing, her enthusiasm, inspiration, good will, and sense of humor all contribute to a sense of fun I would have never thought possible in my early mornings...She not only figured out how to strengthen my back, but also took in stride any sudden re-injury set backs so that I never had to completely stop training. She could always figure out how to lessen the impact and find a work around. It wasn't long before my enthusiasm and results made my more skeptical attorney husband notice and want his own training. Although we have worked with JJ for years now, I still often marvel at her ability to switch her approach to our very different left brain/ right brain styles of learning. It is only in listening to her answer the most detailed questions about why or why not a particular movement or strategy will heal or harm, that you begin to realize the scope and depth of her knowledge and training. Meanwhile subtly, and not so subtly, she has influenced our food choices for healthier eating, and life choices for more positive and spiritual thinking. Her energy and enthusiasm for her own evolution and life's work is contagious making her a wonderful mentor and life coach. She is always an inspiration."

Rose Marie Browning

"I have been working with JJ for going on five years. I first saw JJ present at a workshop and what she said made sense to me. During the time I have been working with her I have found her to be authentic, genuinely interested in my health and well-being and a great support in meeting some of the challenges I have encountered along the way. Not only that but having worked with other trainers in the past, I can say that JJ definitely knows what she is doing. If I have discussed an injury with her she has been able to, without actually seeing me, pinpoint what the problem might be. Later the doctor's diagnosis would often confirm her original opinion. She has also been able to work around injuries, vacations, and adjusts the workouts she gives me to my fitness level and time I have available to workout. She also has worked on my eating habits, which has not been an easy task. Her approach is unique in this aspect and I have made some positive adjustments to my eating. JJ practices what she preaches and is always learning and trying new things. When she believes that something works she shares it with her clients. JJ is a positive thinker and takes an holistic approach. I would recommend her to anyone who is serious about their overall health and fitness."

Christine Hover

"I have been working with JJ Flizanes for many years. Before I started working with JJ, I had never really worked out much. I have played golf, ski and do various outdoor sporting events from time to time but never had formal exercise in my life. Here we are, almost 6 years later and close to 15 lbs lighter, and I can't imagine my life without it. I love feeling strong, having muscle and more energy. Through JJ's training one on one with me in person and over Skype, her podcast and the classes she gives at my company, I have learned how easy it can be to eat better, how stress impacts my body and how important my health really is to me. I can honestly say I have a different relationship with my body than I ever have before."

Greg Lay

After having JJ Flizanes as my life coach, for only two months, I am amazed how much she has inspired me to take the necessary steps to begin healing. JJ's advice, being an expert in so many fields, gave me the courage to peel off many layers to uncover my debilitating core beliefs. Once discovered, she has been teaching me strategies to replace my dysfunctional thoughts and behaviors with techniques to transform myself into a self-loving confidant woman I always dreamed about becoming! I am excited about the endless possibilities with continuing my work with JJ!

Susan Stanton

"After countless trainers I discovered JJ. She has found the key...the key to me. Her passion for fitness is to get me to perform for myself, and the understanding of how my mind and body work in concert. Through her knowledge she has taught me how to manage my stress and the part it plays in my overall health program. I finally learned to let go and let JJ. Amazing results!"

Sharon Tedesco

"After following JJ Flizanes' podcasts and being a client for the past 3 years, I am always amazed and inspired by her vast knowledge of everything needed for living your best happy, healthy life. I can honestly say I look at life differently after working with JJ and being exposed to her holistic approach that includes emotional health. I now have a better understanding of myself, my triggers and a new awareness. What I love is that JJ also has a solution for all it. She truly cares about each and every one of the people she touches and wants us all to live our best lives possible."

Brenda Phillips

"It gives me the greatest of pleasure to let you know that after resisting my wife's pleading over many years to appoint a Personal Trainer for myself I finally caved in and appointed you to take care of my body's many problems such as erratic gait, difficulty climbing stairs, limited movement in both my shoulders, lack of energy in my body, I looked sick, felt it and felt miserable. Only five sessions with you has opened up new chapter in my life. I walk straight, I can run up the stairs and both my arms have painless mobility and greater movement. I have energy in my body, I look 10 years younger and feel it and my mood is cheerful and I like to talk. JJ I can't thank you enough for doing what you did for me and above all it is not even painful and I love doing it. So take this to the bank and cash it. Thanks so much."

Surjit K.

"JJ, Your knowledge, of fitness and nutrition along with your patience just amazes me. You've shown me I can do this, I really didn't think I could. Being diagnosed with RA five years ago, I didn't think I would ever feel in control of my body physically again. I'm still learning to work through it one day at a time but I now know I CAN. Thanks!"

Colleen S.

"My wife has danced and exercised most of her life and has always been in great shape but in the past few months after adding resistance training and using a heart monitor during her aerobic workouts, I have seen some amazing changes in her body. Her endurance and muscle tone has noticeably improved. Her continued commitment to herself through exercise and affirmations has not only helped her but our entire family as well. JJ, Deb looks amazing. I don't think people believe her when she tells them she has had 5 children. Your program was just what she needed to kick her up to the next level. The lucky husband"

Charles W.

"JJ Flizanes is a wealth of knowledge. Her way of coaching truly embodies holistic healing, an understanding that all parts of our lives are connected. She is supportive and nurturing but honest and to the point. The process of losing weight can be so frustrating and overwhelming but having the correct information makes it easy to implement the changes you need to see progress in every aspect! I'm nowhere near perfect, but the most important thing JJ has taught me is that I don't have to be perfect."

Julie Wolfe

"I travel almost every week for work, logging over 150,000 miles in a typical year. About a year ago, I discovered that I have a degenerative hip and that hip replacement surgery is imminent. I was advised by several doctors to put the surgery off as long as I could by strengthening muscles and increasing flexibility in and around the damaged area. During the past year

I visited five doctors, a chiropractor, saw two different physical therapists and started taking pilates. Prior to my injury, I had been going to the gym regularly, alternating between running on the treadmill and doing a spin class. Both became too painful on my hip and I didn't know of any alternative workouts, so I generally just quit going to the gym and gained 10 pounds. JJ has designed a training regimen for me that I can perform while traveling, in my hotel room. During the first month, I lost seven pounds and my hip feels better than it has in the past year. She is a pleasure to work with and I really appreciate the specialized program she designed for me".

Mike B.

"When looking for a personal trainer, I was sort of leery about working out in my home. I thought "How good of a workout could I possibly get at home?" and "How disciplined will I actually be working out at home?" My questions were answered as soon as JJ trained me for my first workout. Boy was I wrong! I didn't know how great of a workout I could get right in my living room! And it's so convenient, right after my workout, I just go upstairs, get a shower and get ready for work! Much better than going to a gym, taking a bag full of clothes/workout gear to and from my car. Last time I did that, the workout bag lived in my car. Thanks to Invisible Fitness, I get a workout that's convenient."

Casey G.

"I have worked with JJ for about 2 years now, and have come to value her opinion highly. She is a holistic person, looking at all parts of your life to improve and make you better. Mind, spirit, body and diet for me! I suffered a bad case of Diverticulitis and had visited many doctors, all with dire thoughts of surgery. JJ was all about healing yourself and how we can help with that. First thing was changing the diet by eliminating anything processed, all dairy and all wheat products. Within a month I knew that dairy was a real issue with me. I had lots of low grade infections on my skin and they all healed in that time. Those same infections were bothering my gut. A year later and I have no symptoms of infection-truly a life changing event for me.

Our exercise program is no less dramatic. I had broken a leg and hip years earlier from a bike accident. It left me with many issues, shorter leg, damaged muscle tissue and a bad foot from walking oddly. She has worked around this, and strengthened my leg, and core so I am stronger and able to hike 5 to 7 miles. I love her approach to workouts. The weights are enough to cause you to fail, but light enough not to damage you either. The focus is always on small groups of muscles, visualizing them as they contract and do the work. This year skiing has been quite incredible with a strong core and legs. I am skiing better than I have in 15 years. Thanks JJ for helping me improve my life!"

Morgan Holt

"Where do I start? Miracles happen! I have lost close to 30 pounds and have regained core strength that has been missing for 20 years!! I have three other family members working with Invisible Fitness (and want a fourth one to start soon), and it has been a true intervention for each one. We are all planning to run a 5K race together in a week, something that we never dreamed possible. The high level of expertise that Invisible Fitness brings to the training process makes the difference between ineffective efforts and tangible, real results! All our thanks to JJ and Invisible Fitness!!"

June H.

"I lost 11 pounds, 6% body fat and 5.5 inches! During the school year, I used to make excuses about how I couldn't fit in exercise and now I commit every week to it and find the time in my schedule that I used to think I didn't have. I also have learned to be more gentle with myself. I would recommend this to people who want to be really honest with themselves and are ready for change. You are very good at what you do! You have helped me in so many ways. I really appreciate everything I have learned and feel great about the results I have gotten. I have more confidence now that I can continue on this path for even more!"

Kristin B

"True story. After a serious lower back surgery, I hadn't worked out in almost two years. Then, out of the blue, I got a reality show where I had to become a Chippendale dancer in less than 8 weeks. Enter JJ and INVISIBLE FITNESS. She showed me how to gain muscle while simultaneously losing fat, all the while protecting and strengthening my back. After 6 weeks of seriously intense training on her cardio, weightlifting and diet program, I not only looked like a Chippendale, I felt like one. I gained 10 pounds of solid muscle in my chest and shoulders, lost all the fat around my belly, and had the fitness to endure 4 hour dance workouts. Thanks JJ!"

Adam W.

"JJ has been a tremendous help in me getting my feminine energy back. I was so depressed and overweight and out of shape and in my masculine energy since my divorce. I had forgotten how to nurture myself as a woman and how to fit myself up with light, love, creativity and joy. She reminds me what it is like to be in a happy marriage that's working. She represents a large part of what I desire in a marriage and she has reminded me that I can and will attract the perfect partner for me once I focus on ME. With JJ's help I am now dancing again! I am getting my sensuality and femininity back again. I am playing soft music in my home for myself and kids. I am taking bubble baths instead of showers, I am walking with a sway in my hips again- thank you JJ"

Echo Allen

"One of the most important things in your lifetime is caring for your child. We got in contact with Invisible Fitness to help our 13 year old son become fit for his football season. Dominic had a great time working with JJ. Not only did she point him in the right direction about eating healthy foods but she did great workouts with him to develop his muscles all the while making sure that every step he took with his workout was safe and healthy. It's great to see somebody like JJ truly care for the well-being of your child. JJ's workouts were phenomenal, she was able to communicate well with our young teen and develop great results. As a parent it is truly awesome to see the end result. We now how a strong healthy child that excels on the football field because of his increased speed, strength and self -confident, all a result from his training with Invisible Fitness and JJ Flizanes."

John and Carolyn L.

"Today, my son and I were about to enter the gym when one of the ladies who teaches Group Fitness, who was also entering the gym, said to me, "You must be very proud of yourself." I said, "why's that?" She continued" with how you have transformed your body, you look great." I was shocked. I have to admit that I am surprised on how well coaching over the phone is working. Even with not being able to work together physically, you have gotten me down the better path. The tools you have introduced and the better use of my time with cardio and weights at the gym, as well as the more fruits have really changed my mental being. I have wondered why it's called invisible fitness, now I know why. It starts with the inside and we have all been "trained" by media that the outside is where the priority is. I've been doing the outside for years and now I see it starts inside. The outside will follow suit. You have helped me see things in a much better light, plus put me down the better path. I feel great!! YOU HAVE EVEN MORE TALENT THEN JUST GOOD WORKOUTS. I've been able to keep on the positive side of things-readjusting my thinking, so it's not getting the best of me. My stress level hasn't been there, Thanks JJ, You have the greatest insight. "

Sally M.

"Even with only having been utilizing your services as a personal trainer for three weeks now, I can't tell you how much happier I am to be exercising at home with very little equipment as opposed to traveling to a gym for a workout. By remaining at home it is helping me focus on changing my *lifestyle* instead of just working out. As for the workout, I find that I can concentrate much better on what I'm doing at home, and ideally have a more efficient workout that way. In conclusion, for me the benefits of staying home to exercise are convenience, the big picture of lifestyle change, avoiding a meat market atmosphere, and (this must be stressed again) convenience. Thanks for helping me head back in the direction I've been yearning"

Ken G.

"I have worked with JJ Flizanes on her 90 Day Program. JJ's program, although dealing very much with physical health and well-being also deals with the mental and emotional balance life needs to be complete. I not only feel more fit but I feel very positive in spite of the turmoil and stress that surrounds me. I'm better able to cope with the curve balls. I look forward to the exercise on a daily basis and I crave healthier foods. The weekly phone calls keep me focused and JJ has really helped me to see a long term picture for a fit and fabulously healthy future. I'd recommend this program to everyone, JJ is awesome."

Leah K.

"Investing in work-outs with JJ is a rational way of removing excuses. For me, she worked around shoulder bursitis and an old knee injury; and I know those joints are surrounded and supported by better muscle than before. Obviously she makes the excuse of not liking the gym go away; do not be deceived by her bungee cords and light weights. Using gravity and your own body she can give you a work-out that will push your muscles to their limit."

John O.

"Invisible fitness is a Godsend for me. I have had Multiple Sclerosis for 15 years and have functioned fairly well in spite of needing to use a cane from time to time.(Female Cabaret Artist of the Year for 2003 in Los Angeles) Attitude is everything when it comes to my healing and Invisible Fitness as a company makes that their number one priority and it has totally transformed me. I am actually excited to workout,that right there is some kind of miracle! I don't consider this service a luxury (even though I'm treated like a Queen) for me it's a necessity! It keeps on my feet and singing for my 90 minute one woman shows..."

Deborah D.

"When I hired JJ and Invisible Fitness, I had two goals in mind, the toning up of my body, and my getting back into a 32 inch pair of tuxedo pants from a 34 plus inch waist (I had a wedding date to meet 6 months away). One of JJ's challenges was working with someone that had had back surgery and was prone to back soreness. She has managed to successfully challenge me into realizing my goals. Using hand and leg weights as well as some bungee cords, I have re-developed muscles that I long ago lost. Her goal-setting cardiovascular guidance helped me achieve the weight loss necessary to fit into my tuxedo, all this in a manner that was both healthy and one that I can live with for the rest of my life."

Mark D.

"When my husband told me to go out and buy some sexy lingerie, I knew that my training with Invisible Fitness was really paying off. After two pregnancies, I had about 20 pounds to lose and my lower abs were just not working. With JJ's program, I have gone down two sizes, my abs are now working, and I feel transformed. In the words of my husband when I put on a new smaller outfit for the first time, "JJ is really sculpting you!" JJ and her crew make the training fun, varied, and personalized to my needs; best of all, they produce results. Invisible Fitness is the best."

Lisa P.

"The workshop that JJ presented to our team was fantastic and we all attained great benefit from her wisdom and enthusiasm! Following the workshop, we all received products and programs. This program has made a tremendous difference to me in overall life management and made me more effective across all my roles. In 90 Days, I have lost over 10 pounds, 3% body fat, 5 inches and I went from wearing a 12/14 down to a 10! My injured back feels strong and pain free and I am shocked at how we have rehabilitated my knee- all over the phone and with the 90 Day materials. I can't endorse JJ, Invisible Fitness and the 90 Day Health and Body Makeover Program enough for its structure and holistic approach. It works with my body, family, job and life. I'd recommend this program to everyone!"

Jacqui K.

"I have to tell you that your program was outstanding! I was a little reluctant at first, I have played sports and lifted weights for over thirty years and I was always was taught to give 110% but never had the good training. Well consequently I have ended up with a few injuries over those years. Your program allows me to get a great work out without the pain I get with the other types of training that I do. I am able to work out in my hotel rooms when I travel, which is becoming more and more every day. I learned more from you about my body and the limits in three hours than I have in thirty years of reading and training. I also received nothing but great comments from my team. Thank you again!"

Chip S.

"It's about making a lifestyle change. I was READY to do it and I started on my own but I knew I needed support to make big changes happen to keep me on track and make sure the plan was both long and short term. In 7 weeks, I have lost 27 pounds and 10.5 inches! I like that I am not in the gym, we train at home and the equipment and tools JJ gave me I can use anywhere. My family celebrated at the beach for Thanksgiving and my birthday and this was the best holiday ever I have had in terms of food and exercise. I did my cardio and homework everyday , even on the days we ate for the special occasion and then I got right back on track. In the past, I would have just said " oh well, I will wait til Monday" But I feel better than I ever have and I didn't want to slow down. I am happy with my results thus far but I am in it for the long term and know I will keep being successful every step of the way!"

Rena D.

"As a Pacific Gas and Electric Company Safety Supervisor, and a member of the Power Generation Division Safety Team, I had the opportunity to utilize the services provided by

Invisible Fitness in support of the company's focus on personal accountability. The Power Generation Division's focus was on personal accountability for one's own wellness. Invisible Fitness guided close to one hundred Power Generation Humboldt Bay Power Plant employees through nondestructive personal fitness self-evaluations. While at the onset of the meeting most felt that they were in fairly good physical condition, the self-evaluation process led by JJ Flizanes showed us that there was much room for improvement. This was an eye opening experience that started us in the right direction to increase the general well-being of our employees. We participated in a professional three hour presentation, conducted by an obvious expert in her field that held the full attention of the meeting attendance. At the end of the session each employee had a wellness plan designed for their specific needs. I can recommend without hesitation the services of Invisible Fitness for any wellness improvement endeavor."

W. David Suchar, PG&E

"JJ had her work cut out with me. I hadn't done any exercise at all in over a year and knew I needed someone special to get me out of my rut. I am beyond delighted that I was able to find JJ. Her approach to personal training is unique, in that she manages to wake up even the most resistant muscles, while seeming to be gentle, non-judging and against pain. Her work outs are actually fun! Her deep understanding of how the body really works inspires confidence because she knows how to strengthen the body gradually with real results. Her approach is so PRACTICAL. My body felt much stronger very quickly and I have a whole new outlook about keeping my body strong and toned. I would recommend JJ to anyone. Her method really works!

Winifred M.

"In the past several years I have worked with 3 different personal trainers, and JJ Flizanes definitely is in a higher class than the norm. JJ's wealth of knowledge about how my body is affected by the way in which I do each exercise is just incredible. We are working on maintaining strength and stamina and have added developing body balance. If you want top quality for your body, look no further."

Carli V.

"With rising health care costs and increased focus on performance and productivity from employees, it is definitely an area of concern for industry. JJ Flizanes brings a fresh perspective and new meaning to the terms "working out" and "eating right." JJ not only promotes and reinforces a healthy lifestyle, she showed our employees how to do it, how to empower themselves to be proactive and take personal responsibility in impacting the outcome of their quality of life. Her presentation was not just a "sit-in-your-chair" and listen presentation. JJ had our employees actively engaged and involved in an exercise session. When I saw 200 field employees on the floor following JJ through a series of exercises, it was a true testament to her unique and inspiring approach to have a strong, positive impact with the group. Even those individuals who were apprehensive and resistant before the presentation had nothing but positive comments afterwards. Overall, what you get from JJ Flizanes is compelling, practical applications for any person or organization facing what many would call an "impossible challenge." Thank you JJ for making a difference,

Michael Sparks /PG&E

"JJ has made a wonderful difference in my fitness. While I have been active all my adult life, I am stronger today than I was five years ago even though I am approaching my mid 60s. She taught me to make my workout time much more effective by tuning into what the muscles and joints are doing. I have osteoarthritis in both knees and she continues to find ways to workout safely and effectively. I am convinced that the quality of my aging is so much better. She is very clear that fitness begins with how and what we think in nearly every aspect of life. I give more thought to what my options are now than to what my limitations might be."

Cindi Holt

"I just had to tell you how thrilled I am with my progress since meeting you JJ! I am amazed with the changes I see in my body—it is like another person looking back at me from the mirror. The real me is starting to emerge! I have lost 20 lbs so far and dropped several sizes, going from an uncomfortable size 14 to an 8 or 10 and I know I will achieve my 40 lb weight loss goal. My neck and back problems are improving and I notice that I truly want to eat well and keep up on my exercise now. My whole lifestyle has changed for the better all due to you. What most impresses me is the way you personalize the program for each person. I've worked with trainers before and the experience this time has been totally unlike those in my past. FINALLY, someone understands how to train me without causing injury! You really "get it."

Deborah G.

"I am my own worst critic. I often cannot see past my perceived deficiencies and I become mired in negativity and simply give up hope...that is until I found JJ! I cannot praise her enough for not only being a great trainer, motivator and teacher; but she is also a tremendous supporter. JJ never ceases to amaze me with her dedication and professionalism as well as her guidance inside and outside the gym. JJ isn't simply just a trainer, she's a guru! After only 3 short months, I have not only changed my body, my health and my energy; but I have changed my outlook on life and I have realized that dedicating even a small amount of time to myself, can change my life completely! Thank you JJ for being the "Trainer of Trainers" and a great friend! I would strongly recommend JJ to anyone looking to make a serious change in their lives - she is a consummate pro, passionate about her craft and lots a fun to burn calories with!!

David W.

"JJ is more than a trainer. JJ helped me identify and manage my excuses and impulses. She helped me focus on the reasons why I could make better choices. JJ's program is empowering and helps establish habits that go far beyond the time you work with her. On the 89th day of my 90-day program, I jogged in a 5K, and finished 20 minutes sooner than I had calculated I could! A year before, I stood on the sidelines at this same race and cheered my husband to the finish line. I remember thinking then that there was no way I would ever want to run...much less choose to run in a race. This year, registering for the race was my idea, and I was able to run more of the race than my husband! After 90 days, I dropped from a size 16 down to a size 12 (but I'm almost in a 10!). I lost seven pounds and 11 inches, and I lowered my body fat by 4%! But the biggest improvement is that I am committed to being good to myself. For the first time in my life, I have made my own health a priority"

Renee L.

"It took me 8 years to put on 60 unwanted pounds, and though I know I'll never be a size 4 again, at 40 years old, I would love to be a size 10. After just 8 weeks, I lost 10 pounds, 7.25 inches, and 3.5% body fat. I eat better, I feel better, I sleep better, and I am clearer of mind and more focused. Two things attracted me to JJ over the other trainers I know, first and foremost is that she has a genuine concern about my personal well-being. The second thing that attracted me to JJ, and something that is very important to me, is that JJ comes from a place of science. JJ makes it her business to know the science; why things do what they do and how that will physiologically change and affect you. She educates herself constantly on the cutting edge, latest information, and then she shares it with me, so I am confident that I am getting the absolute best possible training available. Thank you JJ, from the bottom of my scale!"

Diana D.

"For me personally, I experience JJ as a life coach. She shows you how to heal yourself. She shows you how to get stronger. These workouts have changed my workouts from pain to healing. JJ is love. She is very dedicated to helping you. I feel like I am learning HOW to take care of myself, since I started working with JJ. She is a very loving and gentle person. JJ makes me feel she cares and she is full of good information. She understands women's bodies and is a good listener. JJ knows the mind body spirit connection and that is way true healing can take place. It is great to have a person like this in your corner. We all need a coach to put it all together. The most frequent comment I hear is that I now look younger. Did I find the fountain of youth? I believe I did"

Sharon G.

"I am tremendously impressed with the exceptional level of proficiency and knowledge from INVISIBLE FITNESS. The approach to avoid injury first, by focusing on building a solid foundation of fitness in specific areas that are a problem for me is truly wise. I have discovered subtle aspects of posture and motion that are changing me, making me more aware and better able to develop in a wise and healthy way. I recommend and Invisible Fitness and JJ Flizanes."

John O.

ABOUT THE AUTHOR

J J FLIZANES IS AN Empowerment Strategist and the Host of The Fit 2 Love Podcast Show. She is the Director of Invisible Fitness, an Amazon best-selling author of *Fit 2 Love: How to Get Physically, Emotionally, and Spiritually Fit to Attract the Love of Your Life*, and the author of *Knack Absolute Abs: Routines for a Fit and Firm Core*. She was named Best Personal Trainer in Los Angeles for 2007 by Elite Traveler Magazine.

JJ vividly reminds us that the word 'fitness' is not just about the state of one's physical body, but also the factors which determine a person's overall well-being.

For JJ, the key components in all these areas are 'invisible'— balanced support structures of nutrition, emotional centeredness, and health. A favorite of journalists and the media for her depth of knowledge and vibrant personality, JJ, a contributing expert for Get Active Magazine, has also been featured in many national magazines, including *Shape, Fitness, Muscle and Fitness HERS, Elegant Bride,* and *Women's Health* as well as appeared on NBC, CBS, Fox 11, and KTLA. She is also a video expert for About.com and regular contributor for The Daily Love.

JJ launched her professional career in 1996 as the Foundations Director for the New York Sports Club, where she designed curriculum and in-house certification for new and previously uncertified fitness trainers. She has also been certified by the American Council on Exercise (ACE), International Sports Science Association (ISSA), National Academy of Sports

Medicine (NASM), and the Resistance Training Specialist Program (RTS).

With a focus on biomechanics, JJ has lectured for The Learning Annex and as a featured speaker for New York Times Bestselling Author of *The Millionaire Mind*, T. Harv Ecker's *Peak Potentials* seminars, as well as corporate clients, including Pacific Gas and Electric, Hanson Engineering, and Jostens, Inc. She is the Wellness Expert for KFC International and a Fitness Expert for Nourishing Wellness Medical Center.

She has been working in the health and wellness industry for close to 20 years, as a fitness trainer, with a knack for helping her clients become more self-aware and self-empowered through her ability to quickly identify and pinpointing problem areas, and then creating simple solutions involving exercise, nutrition, and mindset changes. She is the Host of the new iTunes Podcast Show Fit 2 Love: Physical, Emotional, and Spiritual Fitness for the Happy Life You Deserve, which is six day a week video and audio show.

What sets JJ apart from her Celebrity Fitness counterparts is the holistic approach to getting results. Over the last fourteen years she has studied, used, and applied Positive Psychology, Neuro-Linguistic Programming (NLP), Eye Movement Desensitization and Reprocessing (EMDR), Emotional Freedom Technique (EFT), Laws of Attraction, Quantum Physics, Non Violent Communication, Imago Therapy, and Hypnotherapy. JJ Flizanes has proven that she's not only an expert in matters of the body and fitness—she's an insightful and provocative author who delivers a timely message about matters of the heart.

RESOURCES & REFERENCES

Nourishing Wellness Medical Center
www.nourishingwellness.com

Dr. Joseph Mercola
www.mercola.com

Entero Labs- Stool Test
https://www.enterolab.com

Weight Loss Resistance Quiz
www.fit2love.tv/quiz

Dr. Lynne Boutross
http://lynneboutross.com

Dr. Elizabeth Plourde
http://www.newvoice.net

Rodger Sorrow, NVC
www.chooseconnection.com

Non Violent Communication
http://www.cnvc.org

Bristol Stool Chart
http://www.bristolstoolchart.net

Tools Listed in Book
www.invisiblefitness.com

The Invisible Fitness Academy
www.invisiblefitnessacademy.com

30 Day Manifestation Challenge
www.fit2love.tv/30daym

Books

If Life is a Game, These are the Rules, Dr. Cherie Carter Scott

Excitotoxins: The Taste That Kills, Dr. Russell Blaylock

Breakthrough: Eight Steps to Wellness, Suzanne Somers

Gifts of Imperfection: Let Go of Who You Think You're Supposed to Be and Embrace Who You Are, Brene Brown

Hysterectomy, Ovary Removal, and Hormone Replacement: What All Women Need to Know , Dr. Elizabeth Plourde

Non Violent Communication: Create Your Life, Dr. Marshall Rosenberg

Your Relationships, and Your World in Harmony with Your Values Messages From The Body: Their Psychological Meaning, Michael J Lincoln, Ph.D

Daring Greatly: How the Courage to Be Vulnerable Transforms the Way we Live, Love and Parent and Lead Brene Brown

Radical Self Forgiveness: The Direct Path to True Acceptance Colin Tipping

Wheat Belly: Lose the Wheat, Lose the Weight, and Find Your Path Back to Health, William Davis, Ph.D

Untethered Soul: The Journey Beyond Yourself Michael A. Singer

Knockout: Interviews with Doctors Who are Curing Cancer Suzanne Somers

Goddesses Never Age: The Secret Prescription, Christiane Northrup, M.D. *for Radiance, Vitality and Well-Being*

The Paleo Diet: Lose Weight and Get Healthy by Eating the Foods You Were Designed to Eat Loren Cordain, Ph.D

Healing Back Pain: The Mind Body Connection
John E. Sarno, M.D.

The Biology of Belief: Unleashing the Power of Consciousness, Matter & Miracles, Bruce H. Lipton, Ph.D

The Unhealthy Truth: One Mother's Shocking Investigation into the Dangers of America's Food Supply-And What Every Family Can Do to Protect Itself, Robyn O'Brien

Anatomy of the Spirit: Seven Stages of Power and Healing
Caroline Myss, Ph.d

Sacred Contracts: Awaken Your Divine Potential
Caroline Myss, Ph.d

The Surrender Experiment: My Journey into Life's Perfections
Michael A. Singer

Proof of Heaven: A Neurosurgeon's Journey into the Afterlife
Eben Alexander, M.D.

You Can Heal Your Life, Louise Hay

Fabulous Forever: A Woman's Guide to Feeling Joyful, Loving and Free, Carol Chanel

Fit 2 Love: How to Get Physically, Emotionally and Spiritually Fit to Attract the Love of Your Life, JJ Flizanes

Knack Absolute Abs: Routines for a Fit and Firm Core
JJ Flizanes

PODCASTS AND VIDEOS

Fit 2 Love: Physical, Emotional, and Spiritual Fitness

For the Happy Life You Deserve
www.fit2love.tv

Smart Exercise: Get Results & Protect Your Joints
www.jjflizanes.com

Easy Paleo, Gluten, & Dairy Free Cooking
www.jjflizanes.com

Nutrition and Alternative Medicine
www.jjflizanes.com

The Emotional Side of Wellness
www.jjflizanes.com

Spirit, Purpose & Energy
www.jjflizanes.com

REFERENCES

Natural Medicines Comprehensive Database Consumer Version. Information from this source is evidence-based and objective, and without commercial influence. For professional medical information on natural medicines, see *Natural Medicines Comprehensive Database Professional Version.* ©

Gaby AR. Dehydroepiandrosterone: biological effects and clinical significance. Alter Med Rev. 1996;1(2):60-9.

American Heart Association. Wald, D. *British Medical Journal*

Wellness Today May 6, 2014

1 Am J Clin NutrMarch 2004 vol. 79 no. 3 362-371

2 The International Society for Clinical Densitometry, Vitamin D Deficiency: The Silent Epidemic of the Elderly

3 American Journal of Geriatric Psychiatry December 2006; 14(12): 1032-1040

4 Mayo Clinic Proceedings June 21, 2013

1 Hemochromatosis.org

2, 3 Irondisorgers.org, Four Important Tests Where Ranges for Normal Vary (PDF)

Medical News Today July 1, 2014

1 Alzheimer›s Association 2011 Alzheimer›s Disease Facts and Figures

2 DrPerlmutter.com

Folate | Linus Pauling Institute | Oregon State University. (2016). Lpi.oregonstate.edu.

10 Journal Of Inherited Metabolic Disease, 34(1), 75-81

Dr. Mark Houston ,the University of Vanderbilt, author of*What Your Doctor May Not Tell You About Heart Disease*

Dr. Russell Blaylock, an oncologic neurosurgeon out of the University of Mississippi *Excitotoxins: The Taste That Kills.*

www.webmd.com

http://www.mercola.com/

Mayoclinic.org